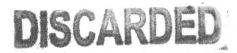

Disorders of Articulation

CHARLES VAN RIPER, editor *Foundations of Speech Pathology Series*

Prentice-Hall Foundations of Speech Pathology Series

PRENTICE-HALL INTERNATIONAL, INC., *London*
PRENTICE-HALL OF AUSTRALIA, PTY. LTD., *Sydney*
PRENTICE-HALL OF CANADA, LTD., *Toronto*
PRENTICE-HALL OF INDIA PRIVATE LTD., *New Delhi*
PRENTICE-HALL OF JAPAN, INC., *Tokyo*

Disorders of Articulation

JAMES A. CARRELL

Professor of Speech
University of Washington

Prentice-Hall, Inc., *Englewood Cliffs, N.J.*

editor's note

THE SET OF VOLUMES WHICH CONSTITUTES THE *Foundations of Speech Pathology Series* is designed to serve as the nucleus of a professional library, both for students of speech pathology and audiology and for the practicing clinician. Each individual text in the series is written by an author whose authority has long been recognized in his field. Each author has done his utmost to provide the basic information concerning the speech or hearing disorders covered in his book. Our new profession needs new tools, good ones, to be used not once but many times. The flood of new information already upon us requires organization if it is to be assimilated and if it is to help us solve the many different professional problems which beset us. This series provides that essential organization.

One of the unifying and outstanding features of all the volumes in this series is the use of search items. In addition to providing the core of information concerning his subject, each author has indicated clearly other sources having significance for the topic being discussed. The reader is urged to explore, to search, and to discover —and the trails are charted. In so rapidly changing a profession as ours, we cannot afford to remain content with what we have been taught. We must learn to continue learning.

Although each individual volume in this series is complete unto itself, the instructor should welcome the opportunity presented by the *Foundations of Speech Pathology Series* to combine several volumes to form the basic structure of the course he teaches. They may also be used as collateral readings. These short but comprehensive books give the instructor a thoroughly flexible teaching tool. But the primary aim of the authors of these texts has been the creation of a basic library for all of our students and professional workers. In this series we have sought to provide a common fund of knowledge to help unify and serve our new profession.

contents

ix

Disorders of Articulation

DISORDERS OF ARTICULATION ARE THE MOST FREQUENT AND POTEN-tially handicapping of all speech disorders. As such, they are the greatest single challenge faced by the speech pathologist. But while they occupy much of his time and tax his ingenuity greatly, they also afford him a rewarding opportunity to contribute significantly to the welfare of those children and adults whose communication is impaired in this way.

This book is concerned with the correction of disorders of articulation. Successful clinical procedures cannot, however, be reduced to any set of prescribed formulas. Instead, they must be developed from an understanding of the nature and etiology of a disorder *and* its unique occurrence in the individual under treatment. For this reason, our approach to articulation training will be through an

1 *general considerations*

attempt to describe systematically the phenomena of defective articulation, the factors which may disrupt the normal articulation process, and those theoretical considerations which underly successful clinical procedures.

THE NATURE OF THE ARTICULATION PROCESS

Articulation is often defined narrowly, either explicitly or by inference, as the "molding" in the mouth of the outgoing breath stream—voiced or unvoiced—into various speech sounds through movements of the "organs of articulation," that is, the muscles in and around the oral cavity. Such definitions treat this component of the articulation process, along with respiration, phonation, and the neurophysiological events that arouse and control the expressive speech movements as separate, although related, aspects of speaking. Disordered articulation, however, is much more comprehensible if articulation is conceived of as a *total* response of the organism in which all elements of these neuromuscular activities are integrated so that speech signals are created and differentiated from one another into meaningful utterance.

Even this broader concept is not completely adequate for interpreting clinical phenomena, since articulation is only one part of the communication process. Speaking is not actually a sequence of separate steps such as reception, symbolization and language formu- **1** lation, respiration, phonation, and "articulation." Instead, these various aspects of communication are interrelated to such a degree that articulation, both normal and abnormal, can be understood only as part of a total response.

> 1   Osgood's (218) conceptual model may clarify the relationship of expressive speech movements to the total process of communication.

Any defect of articulation, then—say a "functional" sound substitution—can result from a breakdown at any number of places in the total process of speaking, so that it is not enough to say that the speaker has made "wrong tongue movements" when, in fact, the misarticulation was an incorrect total pattern of responses. Treatment, of course, should be based on this concept.

Normal and abnormal articulation can be understood only in terms of both structure and function, and the relationship between them. A description of the anatomy and physiology of speech is

> 2   The reader who needs to do so might consult Palmer and LaRusso (220) or Kaplan (152). An excellent summary of the neurological basis of speech is in Eisenson, Auer, and Irwin (77).

outside the scope of this book, but the functional aspects of articulation will be reviewed in terms of (1) activities that take place in what is sometimes called the peripheral speech mechanism, and (2) the neurophysiological antecedents to the speech movements. Of great importance to this discussion will be a review of the way in which articulation responses develop in the child as he is learning to talk, for developmental disorders are perhaps more frequent than those acquired after speech has been established.

Articulation Movements

Speech requires an integrated action of the entire sound-producing and modulating system; the respiratory movements that create breath pulses, the nice adjustments of the laryngeal musculature, and the modulating or differentiating movements of the articulation musculature in and about the mouth make up a single integrated synergic response. Training a person who has defective articulation is an attempt to develop in him such total patterns of response.

An appreciation of the nature of these audible signals is necessary for an understanding of the process of articulation. The analysis of any language from the point of view of structural linguistics leads, in part, to identification of its basic phonetic units, often called *phonemes;* these are the distinctive sound families which, in various combinations, make up the spoken words of the language. When language is written, some set of symbols is employed to represent these sounds. For representing speech as *sound,* a system of notation such as the alphabet of the International Phonetic Association is used, which is less confusing than conventional orthographic symbols.

3 Convenient references for the IPA include Carrell and Tiffany (50), Kenyon and Knott (154), or the section on pronunciation in Webster's *Third New International Dictionary of the English Language* (324). An alternative basis for speech analysis is presented by Trager and Smith (310).

Strictly speaking, however, *phonemes* are linguistic units; they are not the basic physiological or acoustic elements of articulation. A phoneme such as [f], for example, is sometimes described as a *family* of sounds; sounds which fall within any of the basic phonemes are produced with generally similar articulation movements, but there are slight differences among them. These differences in pronunciation do not affect meaning, but they are important for correct articulation. The sounds which fall within any of the phonemes are termed *allophones* of the phoneme in question. Sounds within any of the phonemes are perceived as the "same" sound; sounds from different phonemes are perceived as "different" sounds. [f] and [k], for instance, represent different phonemes since even the untrained listener hears them as distinctively different. The choice of [f] or [k] as a final sound determines whether one says "laugh" or "lack"; hence, meaning is affected. Again, "fuss" [fʌs] and "fuzz [fʌz] convey different ideas because of the variation in the final sounds; [s] and [z] therefore differ phonemically.

4 Carrell and Tiffany (50) have undertaken a further discussion of phonemes and allophones in terms suited to the interests of the speech correctionist.

In *speaking* there are no exact physiological counterparts for these linguistic units; the basic units of articulation, insofar as any can be distinguished, are of a different kind. When samples of ongoing speech are analyzed by careful laboratory techniques it is usually impossible to fix any definite boundaries between phonemes. For instance, if one were to inspect a spectrographic record of the spoken word "tea," he could not point with any confidence to the exact place where [t] leaves off and [i] begins; the two sounds blend into a unique configuration. The *syllable* is therefore generally regarded as the irreducible unit of speaking, and it is often the unit of remedial training in articulation disorders. Under some circumstances, even the boundaries between syllables cannot be located exactly. For example, a dividing point between the first and second syllabic pulses in "football" might be relatively easy to define, but this would not be true of the two-syllable utterance, "push him" [puʃ ɪm].

> 5   Anyone not thoroughly familiar with the concept of the syllable should consult either McDonald (180) or Carrell and Tiffany (50). Stetson (292) is an original source.

Articulation is a process in which there is a constant flow and flux of neuromuscular adjustments with parallel acoustic signals. Speech is not the utterance of a series of separable sounds or even syllables, although such sounds and syllables can be distinguished from a linguistic point of view. Traditional phonetic theory recognizes the physiologically and acoustically fluctuating nature of ongoing speech in the concepts of *phonetic influence* and *assimilation,* that is, when sounds are combined in the configurations of speaking they change from what they might have been, had it been possible to utter them in isolation. This stress on the differences between speech as a linguistic phenomenon and speech as a physiological and acoustic phenomenon has a direct bearing on the methods of speech correction that will be recommended in a later chapter.

Antecedents to Articulation Movements

The highly complicated neuromuscular responses of articulation, perhaps the most intricate of all forms of human motor behavior, obviously could not operate without correspondingly elaborate neurological control systems. Our treatment of this complex subject, which is still incompletely understood in some particulars, must necessarily be schematic and in terms of function.

> 6   Kaplan (152) covers the basic facts of neurophysiology with which one should be familiar for an understanding of the neurogenic disorders of articulation.

The term *antecedents* to articulation movements stands for all those aspects of neurophysiological function that underly the muscular responses that create the speech signal. In one way or another, these antecedents involve complex circuitry in the brain which is programmed so that the patterned movements for meaningful speech can be aroused and the necessary muscular responses executed. Although we must bear in mind that articulation is a total unified process, two aspects of the motor phase of speaking can be identified: (1) a primary motor effector system and (2) motor integrative circuitry.

The primary motor effector system

Articulation movements are mediated by a flow of nerve impulses to those muscles which produce and modulate the sounds of speech. These impulses arrive at the muscles through a *lower motor neuron* network comprised of branches from certain cranial nerves whose nuclei (or point of origin) lie in the *bulbar* portion of the brainstem, and whose peripheral fibers insert into the articulation musculature. This portion of the system is, so to speak, the final common pathway over which are routed the nerve impulses which excite the speech movements. A pathology at this point can impair articulation movements in two possible ways: (1) complete destruction of the nucleus or peripheral fibers of any nerve will result in complete loss of movement and tone in the muscles that nerve serves; or (2) partial destruction of the nucleus or peripheral fibers will result in weakness of motion and a reduction of muscle tone. The effect on speech may range from complete loss of articulation movements to weakness of motion. The term *lower motor neuron dysarthria* can be used for conditions of this kind.

Above the lower motor neuron system (i.e., rostral to the bulbar portion of the brainstem) lies an exceedingly intricate group of neural networks which act to coordinate the action of the complex and rather widely separated muscle groups which are involved in articulation. Without this control of the lower motor system, properly timed and ordered speech movements would be impossible. Three major systems are commonly differentiated at this level, the *pyramidal, extra-pyramidal,* and *cerebellar* pathways. Except in certain special cases, pathology in this portion of the motor circuitry causes a disorder of motion, rather than weakness or an absence of motion. The dysarthrias associated with cerebral palsy fall into this category, and may be of the *spastic, athetoid,* or *ataxic* type.

---

7   McDonald (181), in the volume of this series on cerebral palsy, discusses these matters in further detail, or for a full technical treatment, consult Woodburne (346).

The motor integrative circuitry

At the highest level of the nervous motor system are those circuits laid down through learning for the arousal and control of the muscular responses through which we use language expressively in speaking (and writing). Consideration of this matter would lead to the whole question of the neurophysiological basis for motor learning, which we cannot explore. Certain hypotheses, however, help to explain normal function and some of the acquired and developmental disorders in the articulation process. Essentially, learning a pattern of articulation movements depends on a kind of *programming* of the brain in such a way that *engrams* are laid down, through learning, for the expressive speech movements.[1] Where there is dysfunction of the central nervous system, a child may, apart from mental retardation, be physiologically incapable of forming these memory traces; also, brain damage acquired by older individuals who have learned language normally may cause them to lose the ability to execute the movements for the expressive use of language in speaking or writing. The terms *developmental apraxia* and *acquired apraxia* may be applied to these conditions, or they may be referred to generally as forms of *central dysarthria.*

> 8   A more detailed treatment of apraxia will follow in Chapter 7, but
> some preliminary reading in either Brain (35) or Morley (200) might be
> helpful at this point.

The exact pathways and brain areas which serve this higher motor integrative function cannot yet be identified with any real degree of certainty; indeed, the entire subject of the neural basis of speech and language behavior remains obscure despite the extensive literature available. We must speak with even less confidence about

> 9   Historical summaries of scientific thinking about brain function in rela-
> tion to speech and language can be found in a number of places.
> Head (118) or Schuell (263) are excellent references. Some of the
> experimental evidence reported by Penfield and Rasmussen (223) and
> Penfield and Roberts (224) is of great interest.

the manner in which the engrams for articulation are laid down in the course of an infant's speech development, although certain assumptions can be made.

> [1] In this context, an *engram* is the "trace" or neurological analog for a given pattern of movement which is stored in the brain. Engrams consist of some change in the protoplasm of the brain produced by learning. They constitute a kind of *memory bank* for the execution of learned movement. The term *ekphorize* is sometimes used to refer to the arousal of an engram.

The developmental sequence through which an infant passes in the acquisition of articulation skills seems quite well established. During the early weeks vocalization is reflexive and quite undifferentiated. It is probably derived largely from the neural circuits for feeding movements and other innate reflexes. The musculature which will later be used for articulation is exercised somewhat, but other than that no specific foundation for speech is laid down in these early weeks. At about six weeks, a period of *vocal play* and *babbling* begins, in which the child shows more complex sound-making behavior and more *differentiation* of movement, in contrast to the more generalized reflexive vocalizations. Sounds produced during this period are still to be regarded as derivatives of chewing, suckling, and swallowing movements. This behavior strengthens muscles and lays the groundwork for a rudimentary control of articulation movement, but there is too little specific reinforcement of any particular sounds to support the hypothesis that engrams for articulation are being laid down during the first weeks of babbling.

In the weeks that follow, however, the infant will produce certain patterns of sound more regularly, and some of them will resemble speech sounds of the language environment. As early as the third month the child shows signs of social behavior by responding to speech with sound-making, and shortly thereafter the sounds he babbles begin to be more nearly limited to those of the language spoken around him. He has now entered a stage in which we can infer that specific memory traces for the articulation of the sounds in his language are being acquired. During the interval from the sixth or seventh to the twelfth month the infant produces increasingly more complicated patterns of sound—doubled syllables, true disyllables, and thereafter the familiar jargon of the next stage of speech development. Inflectional and stress patterns like those in the language environment are established, and the foundation is laid for the intricate motor behavior which characterizes connected speech.

10   This discussion is limited to certain aspects of motor development. Morley (200) can be consulted for a more complete description of speech development.

The formation of the engrams for articulation is therefore characterized by progressive differentiation and increasing specificity in the acquisition of the speech sounds. The basic units in which language is learned are not, of course, individual sounds but some unit of that language, possibly *morphemes,* words, or even larger lan-

guage *gestalten.* Assuming for purposes of discussion that words are
the basic unit, as seems likely, it follows that during the learning
process complex neural circuitry must be laid down for arousal of
articulation movements for words, and also for the even more complicated motor responses needed to combine words into the patterns
of connected speech. We may assume this to be a kind of integrative circuitry at the highest level comparable to that which
operates in *language formulation* where, for propositional speech,
words are sequenced and appropriately altered in form according
to the rules of grammar and syntax. Failure in this latter function
leads to some of the manifestations of *syntactic dysphasia.* In a similar way we may hypothesize that some of the subtle disorders of
articulation—to which the terms *apraxia* or *central dysarthria* seem
applicable—represent a comparable defect in the integration of these
higher motor responses involved in articulation.

Receptive Factors

Up to this point we have discussed only the production of articulatory movements. However, all coordinated neuromuscular responses
depend on combined input-output circuitry, for sensory impulses
are indispensable to the control of movement. For example, sensory
tracts leading from certain end organs in the inner ear provide information about the position of the body in space, leading to the
arousal of reflexes which aid in maintaining posture and balance.
Kinesthesis provides information about the direction and extent of
muscular movement, and is necessary for motor control. If sensory
mechanisms do not function normally, as in certain inner ear or
spinal cord diseases, the patient will be unable to maintain posture
or execute coordinated movements normally. If central motor circuitry is impaired, as in cerebellar ataxia, essentially the same symptoms will follow. When the total sensorimotor system is functioning
normally, however, the reverberating circuits operate as a monitoring or "quality control" network to assure coordinated movement.
Learned movements will be carried out as they were learned; reflex
movements will conform to inborn engrams.

Current interest in *cybernetics,* which likens the human nervous
system to an electronic computer, has led to the concept of speech
as a kind of *servosystem* or *servomechanism* in which input-output
feedback loops are the central feature of the basic control mechanisms for articulation. Thus, sensory input information—primarily auditory, kinesthetic, and tactile—aroused by the act of

speaking, is used by error-sensitive *corrector* mechanisms within the brain to maintain the fidelity of the motor responses of articulation. This conceptual model has proved to be a satisfactory approach to articulation-learning theory and for interpretation of both normal and defective articulation. It also provides a rationale for certain methods of training outlined in Chapter 7.

11   Mysak has developed these ideas in detail in his book, *Speech Pathology and Feedback Theory* (209).

To learn articulation, the infant must have normal sensitivity to auditory, kinesthetic, and tactile stimuli. He must first of all hear speech in his environment in order to learn to talk, and the self-stimulation provided by babbling and vocal play is vital in establishing the feedback loops. As he plays with the sounds of speech and later, when he learns to combine them into words, other sensory modalities become important. He unconsciously learns to feel the articulation movements through kinesthesia and through the tactile stimuli of the tongue, lip, and palate surfaces in contact with each other and stimulated by breath flow. These afferent stimuli, integrated at higher levels, thus become incorporated into the feed-

12   Allport (6) has a classical description of this aspect of speech development.

back loops. The importance of the various sense modalities changes as articulation becomes habituated. Audition, which is most critical at the outset, becomes somewhat less important than kinesthesis and touch after speech is well-established, although disturbances in auditory feedback will still impair articulation.

13   Van Riper and Irwin (320) develop these ideas further.

Some final observations should be made about the relationship between the sensorimotor circuits for articulation and the symbolic and semantic aspects of language. One who uses language has, of course, a memory bank in which are stored the engrams for whatever vocabulary he has acquired. The normal brain is programmed so that, when language is formulated and expressed, articulation (or writing) movements appropriate to the symbols can be aroused. Various disorders of the higher language processes may occur when these associative connections are disrupted by brain damage or cannot be learned because of impaired physiological function of the brain. Adults with brain damage, for example, may retain a verbal symbol in every respect save for the capacity to execute correctly (or at all) the appropriate expressive movements (*apraxia*). Children may exhibit a comparable inability to acquire articulation responses without any significant impairment in other language processes.

An interesting sidelight, which has some implications for the neural organization for communication, is that adults with acquired brain damage may retain perfectly normal patterns of articulation, but without appropriate or meaningful verbal content. Children with certain kinds of intellectual defect may likewise have entirely normal execution of motor patterns for speech in the face of severe limitation of verbal capacity. Some, on the basis of *echolalia* or rote memory, can use large numbers of correctly articulated words without any conceptual grasp of what they are saying—a kind of function not unlike that of a tape recorder which receives, stores up, and plays back language which it does not understand.

CRITERIA

Anyone who accepts the responsibility for diagnosis and the planning of treatment must have in mind a clearly formulated set of criteria for defective articulation, insofar as this is possible. This is not a simple matter, for there is in fact no single standard that can be applied in all cases. *Defective* is strictly a working term which, in this context, implies that an individual so labeled is not functioning adequately in those communicative situations he faces or will need to face. There is no abstract standard of good speech. Recognition of this fact is most important in planning goals for training.

The definitions of defective speech in the current literature are generally similar, although they differ somewhat in details. Van Riper (318) regards speech as defective when it calls unfavorable attention to itself, interferes with communication, or causes the speaker to be maladjusted; these characteristics he condenses into the adjectives *conspicuous, unintelligible,* and *unpleasant.* The definition suggested by Berry and Eisenson (26) which is also widely taught, contains much the same criteria. These authors list eight possible characteristics which may mark defective speech: (1) it is not easily audible, (2) it is not readily intelligible, (3) it is vocally unpleasant, (4) it contains specific sound errors, (5) it is labored, or lacks normal inflection or rhythm, (6) it is linguistically deficient,

(7) it is inappropriate to the age, sex, or physical development of the speaker, and (8) it is visibly unpleasant.

> 14   Compare the definitions of defective speech given by Van Riper (318), Berry and Eisenson (26), Johnson, Darley, and Spriestersbach (148), West, Ansberry, and Carr (331), and any others that can be found.

Any of these definitions will probably do well enough as a general guide to diagnosis, but one must not underestimate the difficulty of applying any standard set of criteria to all cases. The diagnostician must also be keenly aware of the risk that his judgments may be too subjective, since there are still only a few genuinely objective criteria, in the laboratory sense, which can be readily applied in a clinic. He should formulate a rational standard in which personal tastes play as little part as possible. Above all other considerations is whether or not the patient, taking into account all the elements of his unique circumstances, has a significant communication disability which is likely to handicap him now or later.

> 15   For some interesting remarks on the larger philosophical question of what constitutes the "normal," consult Johnson, Darley, and Spriestersbach (148).

CLASSIFICATION AND ETIOLOGY

Disorders of articulation can be placed in three categories: (1) *dyslalia,* or those of *functional* origin, (2) *dysglossia,* or disorders referable to an *orofacial* defect, and (3) *dysarthria,* or those which are neurogenic, i.e., arising from some central nervous system pathology which impairs motor speech function. Some writers include a fourth category, *dysaudia,* which includes disorders of articulation secondary to hearing loss, but these are treated as forms of dyslalia in the present text. Some of the literature makes no distinction between dyslalia and dysglossia.

Actually, nomenclature in speech pathology is not well-established, which is unfortunate considering the importance of precise terminology in any field. Consequently, variant usage of terms is to be expected in speech pathology literature. Terms which have some common currency and appear to have reasonably uniform definitions will be introduced at appropriate points in the later discussions.

16   Robbins (242) has edited a dictionary of terms in speech pathology,
      and many of the commoner terms are also listed in a glossary compiled
      by Wood (343). See Ogilvie (215) also.

Distinctions among dyslalia, dysglossia, and dysarthria have value, of course, but there are some subtle difficulties in classifying disorders which can, if they are not recognized, confuse one's thinking both clinically and theoretically. Clinically, a "pure" dysarthria or dysglossia, in which only neurological or structural causes were operative, does not exist. If nothing else, the existence of defective speech, no matter what the cause, will lead to overlaid functional reactions in the speaker. Most articulation disorders seen clinically have multiple causes. Consequently, it is preferable to think in terms of neurological, morphological, and functional *factors* in the etiology of defective articulation. If a given speaker's disorder must be placed in a single nosological category, it is best classified on the basis of what seems to be the *predominating* cause.

17   Rehabilitation Codes, Inc., 1860 Broadway, New York City 10023, is
      developing a coding system which will enable the user to record in
      concise form a variety of etiological and other data about individual
      cases. The code contains a section on communication disorders.

Some clarification is necessary for the term *functional* as it is used in the literature on speech disorders. Medically, a condition is considered functional if there is no demonstrable pathological involvement of an organ system. In speech pathology, a disorder is described as functional if the best diagnostic study that can be made fails to disclose any organic pathology as an antecedent. This does not, however, preclude the possibility that some unknown organic factor has caused the disturbance in function. Furthermore, some theorists argue that any abnormality in function must have an organic analog. Many functional articulation disorders are associated with perceptual defects, learning disabilities, and other deficits which one assumes have some basis, however obscure, in the physical organism. One must also consider that naive or careless diagnosticians may identify problems as functional simply because they have not found observable motor disabilities, orofacial defects, or central nervous system dysfunction that are clearly causative. Clinical applications of these remarks will be made at the beginning of Chapter 3.

18   The foregoing remarks are based in part on comments by Chaiklin and
      Ventry (57) in the course of their discussion of functional hearing loss.
      Compare their point of view with that of Powers (230).

DISORDERS OF ARTICULATION CAN BE STUDIED SIMPLY IN TERMS OF THE errors as they are heard by the listener, quite apart from what may have caused them, hence the speech pathologist should be thoroughly familiar with their phonetic characteristics. The speech pathologist's task is to help the patient learn new and acoustically acceptable speech patterns, and he is concerned with etiology only to the extent that underlying causes may have to be treated before the individual can learn new articulation responses.

Certain etiologies, such as motor disability or hearing loss, usually call for special training methods; on the other hand, the procedures for correcting most articulation disorders have much in common. Moreover, although many causes carry with them characteristic misarticulations, it is also true that different speakers may sound much

2 *phonetic characteristics*

the same, yet have disorders whose etiology is not at all the same.

One should realize that the errors of any given speaker will be unique to him, at least in fine detail, even though there are certain patterns of misarticulation that are broadly similar in many different speakers. Any sound can be misarticulated in so many ways that listing them would be impossible. To cite only one example, a common error in children is an infantile *r* in which [ɝ] and [ɚ] are replaced by a vowel which lacks the "*r*-coloring" of these sounds in General American speech. If one listens to a series of speakers with *r* defects, he will hear a variety of subtle variations in the nonstandard sound. These variations should be noted in a careful phonetic analysis.

> 19 No completely satisfactory system of phonetic notation has been developed for recording such fine individual variations (and probably none ever will be), but the modifying marks used for *narrow transcription* help somewhat. For a description of these see Carrell and Tiffany (50).

The errors committed by a particular speaker are not necessarily consistent. A sound may be misarticulated in one word, but not in another; it may be misarticulated differently from one time to the next even in the same phonetic context. In different phonetic contexts, of course, the errors may vary considerably. For example, [s] might be produced correctly when it is an initial sound (as in *see*), but not when it falls in another position, or is part of **13** a *consonant cluster* or *blend* (as in *sleep, straw,* or *ghost*). The more complicated the articulation adjustment, the greater the likelihood of misarticulation. Inconsistency, however, is so great that no invariable rule can be stated.

There are still other variables. Many speakers habitually mispronounce a given sound, yet can produce it in isolation or even in a word if a model is given for imitation. This is so common that one routinely tests the speaker's ability to imitate when the sounds are spoken for him in isolation, in words, and in contextual speech. Speed of utterance will of course affect the frequency of errors, a fact which must be taken into account in teaching. Finally, the conditions of speaking have a great influence on the number and kind of misarticulations. One may have a *set* which leads to correct speech in one situation, but causes errors in another; he may read aloud correctly, but make errors on the same words in spontaneous speech. Any speech correctionist can remember children who did well during the training session, but called back "dood bye" as they left. Occasionally, pressures can provide motivation which leads to better speech, but the reverse is more often the case. Emotional tensions, confusion in thinking, insecurity, or any other kind of stress may cause marked deterioration in articulation.

> 20   Milisen (194) has developed these points in some detail in connection with methods of articulation testing.

We can turn now to a more specific description of the phonetic characteristics of defective articulation. There is no completely logical way to classify errors, but for convenience they will be placed in the following categories: (1) *phonemic errors,* in which the production of speech sounds has not developed correctly and (2) *configurational* and *contextual* errors, in which the defect is primarily an inability to structure or sequence speech sounds into the word and phrase patterns of normal speech, including abnormalities in the *prosodic* aspects of articulation (rate, pitch melody, and stress). The two kinds of errors may both be present in any speaker, of course, but one may be heard without the other.

PHONEMIC ERRORS

A common type of phonemic error is the *sound substitution,* heard with particular frequency among children with *infantile speech.* Such a child may, for instance, substitute a kind of [w] for [r], so that he seems to be saying "wed" instead of "red." He might have compensated for the missing [r] by saying "-ed" for "red," but we have chosen to consider this kind of phonetic lapse as a configurational error for reasons that will be mentioned later. *Distortions* differ from what we have termed *sound substitutions* only in that they consist of the substitution of a nonstandard rather than a standard sound for the one which would have been correct. The underlying mechanism is the same, although the distorted sound will usually be more nearly correct than the substituted sound.

21   These matters are treated in much greater depth by Van Riper and
      Irwin (320). The present treatment should be reinforced by a study of
      their material on symptomatology.

Phonemic errors occur in a variety of clinical conditions. Major categories include (1) developmental delay in the acquisition of speech skills; (2) sensory and perceptual deficits, including particularly sensory hearing loss and perceptual disabilities associated with brain damage; (3) congenital and acquired orofacial deformities; (4) such cultural factors as foreign and regional dialect, and immediate environmental influences; (5) motor deficiencies, and (6) emotional factors. The reasons why articulation may be defective in these various conditions are reserved for later discussion, but the phonemic misarticulations associated with each are described in the following paragraphs.

Developmental Delay

Infantile speech (called *pedolalia, infantile perseveration* or, in lay terms, "baby talk") is a quite uniform group of phonemic errors, and the commonest of all articulation disorders among preschool and elementary school children. In general, these misarticulations are the result of a developmental delay in the child's acquisition of phonetic skills, which causes him to retain patterns of speech that would be considered normal at an earlier stage of development. Speech containing such phonetic errors after the child has passed his eighth birthday must certainly be considered defective, although it is often prudent to deal with them well before this time.

Studies of the way in which normal children acquire the sounds of speech shed considerable light on this form of delayed development. Despite disagreement on some relatively minor details, these studies show that normal children perfect their use of the speech sounds in a quite uniform order. Vowels and diphthongs (the *syllabic* sounds) are mastered early enough to make their misarticulation infrequent in infantile speech. On the other hand, certain *nonsyllabic* consonant sounds appear relatively late in the developmental order; certainly they are the last to become stabilized as a functional part of the child's repertoire of sounds. These difficult sounds include the *r*-family, [r], [ɝ], and [ɚ] and [s], [z], [θ], [ð], [ʃ], [ʒ], [tʃ], and [dʒ].

Erroneous production of this group of sounds accounts for a large proportion of the typical infantilisms. If these or other sounds are not mastered by the time the child has an expressive word vocabulary of some size, the missing sounds are likely to be replaced by others which he has learned—leading to the typical infantile substitutions. Errors on *r* sounds are a good example of the misarticulations that arise in this way, since this group of sounds is the last to be learned and stabilized in the speech of most children. The nonsyllabic [r] is usually replaced by a labial glide resembling [w], yielding "wabbit," for "rabbit." Many of the sounds which are "avoided" through substitution may have been practiced extensively in vocal play, but were not incorporated into speech. For instance, even though [d] and [g] are generally heard in the average child's speech by the third birthday, the substitution of [d] for [g] ("do" for "go") is a common infantilism—but so also is [g] for [d] ("goggies" for "doggies"). [θ] and [s] are often confused in a similar way, each being substituted for the other, sometimes in the speech of the same child.

22   An older study by Poole (228) is a standard work on the development of speech sounds in the infant. Compare her findings with those of Templin, Irwin, and others to whom reference is made in the bibliography prepared by Johnson, Darley, and Spriesterbach (148).

Certain other trends in the typical errors of infantile speech should be noted. A fact that has considerable clinical importance is that the sounds involved in each of the common infantile substitutions are difficult to discriminate. Many of them (but not all) are relatively hard to hear and identify because, as uttered by the average speaker, they have relatively little acoustic energy. Broadly speaking, syllabics have relatively high and nonsyllabics relatively low acoustic energy. Examples of sounds which are comparatively inaudible are [θ], [f], [s], and [ʃ]; their voiced counterparts, [ð], [v], [z], and [ʒ], carry a greater total amount of physical energy, but not in the frequencies that are critical for their recognition. It is not surprising, then, that the sounds in this group are often confused with one another. Among the sound substitutions which are probably the result of such influences are [f]/[θ] ("fink" for "think"), and [s]/[ʃ] ("soo" for "shoe"), and a number of others.

Many of the sounds that are confused in infantile speech have characteristics which would presumably make them hard to discriminate apart from general audibility. Voiced sounds are substituted for other voiced sounds, plosives for plosives, fricatives for fricatives, and so on. The exceptions to this rule are rare when the articulation disorder is caused by delayed maturation of phonetic skills. It is interesting to note how often, when two sounds are apparently not discriminated, the one whose movements for articulation are more visible is chosen as a substitute for the sound that is less visible. The interchange of [w]/[r] and [f]/[θ] provide excellent examples of this point.

23 Studies of the acoustic characteristics of the various speech sounds, made in the course of perfecting our present telephone system, and reported in part by Fletcher (88), provide an interesting basis on which to analyze possible auditory factors in the sound substitutions of infantile speech.

Following are notes on the sounds most frequently misarticulated in infantile speech:

r-family errors

These include first the substitution of [w] for [r], which is perhaps the most common of all infantilisms. Sometimes this consists of replacing [r] with a standard sound from the [w] phoneme, but often the substituted sound more closely resembles a nonstandard labialized glide which is difficult to represent phonetically, and which varies somewhat from one speaker to another; often the sound in question has a trace of *r* resonance. Occasionally the substitution of [j] (another glide) for [r] is heard. Another *r*-family error is the substitution of a vowel without *r*-coloring for the stressed and unstressed *r*-colored vowels [ɝ] and [ɚ]. There is considerable variation in the sounds that are substituted, but usually they are some variety of central or back vowel. Parents often remark that such children "sound like Southerners" because of the superficial resemblance of their pronunciation to the dialect of that region. Defects of the *r*-family of sounds are the most frequent and persistent of all the developmental deficiencies in phonetic learning, except perhaps for certain forms of lisping. The term *rhotacism* is sometimes applied to any *r* defect.

24   An older text by Nemoy and Davis (212) is still an excellent reference
      on consonant misarticulations and their correction.

Sibilant sound defects

The English *sibilants* include [s], [z], [ʃ], and [ʒ], and any mis-articulation of one or more of these sounds is considered a form of *lisping*. The term *sigmatism* is sometimes used as a synonym for lisping, but is more properly applied only to [s] defects. There is a wide variety of lisping conditions, not all of which can be attrib-uted to developmental delay in phonetic learning. The sibilant sounds are particularly vulnerable to structural deviations in the front part of the mouth. Considering the nature of the lisps that are typical of infantile speech, it seems likely that confusions aris-ing from faulty auditory discrimination are the most likely cause, although difficult articulation adjustments are also required for these sounds. What suggests that faulty discrimination is a major cause of this form of lisping is that the reverse substitutions, [s]/[θ] and [z]/[ð], are by no means unusual among children whose pho-netic maturation is slow. Perhaps the most common infantile lisp is the substitution of [θ]/[s] ("thee" for "see") and [θ]/[z] ("thoo" for "zoo"). This error is variously called a *protrusion, frontal,* or *sub-stitutional* lisp.

Another sibilant defect frequently associated with infantile speech is the *lateral lisp*, although it is also found in speakers with certain kinds of dental malocclusions and in those with the "tongue thrust" habit which will be described later. In its simplest form, a lateral lisp is the substitution of a nonstandard sibilant-like sound made, as the name suggests, with lateral rather than frontal emis-sion of the breath stream. It resembles the fricative that can be made by placing the tongue in the approximate position for [l], then emitting a voiceless breath stream. The resulting sound is acoustically unpleasant when used in a context where [s] is cus-tomarily heard, and is particularly obtrusive when, as so often happens, it is accompanied by the rattle of saliva in the mouth. Some speakers with lateral lisps bring the tongue tip into contact with the alveolar ridge or the anterior part of the hard palate; others do not, but the tongue is nevertheless held in such a way as to obstruct the forward breath flow and force it into lateral channels on either side. Sometimes the tongue is thrust forward to one side or the other of the midline of the upper arch. Although lateral lisping is most common on [s], it is also heard as a defect of [z], [ʃ], [ʒ], and of the *affricates* [tʃ] and [dʒ] as well. Some speakers may lateralize all of these sounds.

Still another variety of lisp, for which the term *occluded* or *occlusion lisp* is sometimes employed, approximates the substitution of [t] for [s] and [d] for [z] and, less often, of [t] for [ʃ] and [d] for [ʒ]. Examples of this form of misarticulation are "tee" for "see" or "titter" for "sister." If one listens to this error closely he will note that the [t] and [d] used as substitutes do not always correspond exactly to standard sounds. For some reason of which the writer is unaware the occlusion lisp seems paːticularly common among children who ultimately prove to have either sensory hearing disabilities or auditory perceptual disorders. Another misarticulation which is quite frequent, but for which no special term has been coined, is the [h]/[s] substitution—as in "hee" for "see."

Poor discrimination among the sibilants is associated with several other errors heard particularly in cases of developmental delay but also in others. Among these errors are [s]/[ʃ] and [z]/[ʒ] substitutions, as in "soo" for "shoe" and "mezer" for "measure." Another is the substitution of [ʃ] for [tʃ], so that "chicken" approximates "shicken." Distorted or nonstandard sibilants in addition to those already mentioned are heard quite frequently, although these are not peculiar to infantile speech. Some speakers produce diffuse "hishing" sounds which are not acoustically identical to lateralized sounds. Sibilants may also be underarticulated and weak, or they may, in contrast, be *strident* or whistling, particularly in the case of [s]. Replacement of [s] by a glottal stop [ʔ] is sometimes noted.

25　A summary and diagramatic representation of the forms of lisping is presented by Van Riper and Irwin (320).

Other fricative misarticulations

Several other errors involving *fricative* sounds are characteristic of infantile speech. Very common is the substitution of [f] for [θ] and [v] for [ð], as in the pronunciation "fink" for "think" and "vat" for "that." A similar misarticulation is an [h]/[θ] substitution, giving such results as "hink" for "think." Children who use this substitution may also replace other voiceless fricatives with [h] ("I hink ho" for "I think so"). Once more acoustic similarity among the sounds appears a likely factor in these errors.

Misarticulation of plosives

These make up another group of the typical errors of infantile speech. Most common of all are the [t]/[k] and [d]/[g] substitutions, yielding pronunciations such as "tap" for "cap" and "det" for "get." Also frequent is the use of a glottal stop [ʔ] in place of [t], [d], [k], and [g] particularly, but also sometimes for [p] and [b] as well. The glottal stop itself has as its major feature a momentary cessation of breath flow or "catch" brought about by arresting movements of the glottis and the musculature of exhalation. A kind of "click" is sometimes perceptible. The acoustic characteristics of a glottal stop are hard to describe verbally, but one may approximate the sound by holding his breath for the briefest of intervals instead of producing [t] in such a word as "water." Occasionally a child with severe phonetic delay is encountered who uses glottal stops so freely as substitutes for plosives and other sounds that superficially his speech seems to consist almost entirely of undifferentiated grunting sounds.

Misarticulations of [l]

Common errors on this sound are its replacement by [w] or [j] in the initial position, the substitution of a sound approximating [w] within words, and the substitution of a central or back vowel (often one which is nonstandard) in the terminal position. Thus, "look" becomes "wook" or "yook" ([jʊk]); "yellow" becomes something like "yewow," and "little" becomes "littuh" or "yittuh." At times the [w] replacing an initial [l] is close to a standard labial glide, but in other cases careful analysis will disclose that the speaker is producing what might best be described as a *labialized* [l]—a sound made with lip rounding, but which retains at least some [l] resonance. There is wide variation in the vowels which take the place of a final [l], but for the most part they have the quality of central or back vowels. The term *dark* [l] (produced with tongue retraction) is sometimes used in this connection, although this same sound may also replace initial and medial [l] sounds. A vowel/final [l] substitution is often heard incorrectly as an omission. The term *lambdacism* has been coined for [l] misarticulations, but is rarely used.

Misarticulation of affricates

Substitutions for the affricate sounds [tʃ] and [dʒ] are frequent in infantile speech. Probably the most common is [ʃ]/[tʃ] ("shicken" for "chicken"), but the substituted sound may be [h], an approximation of [ts], or even a glottal stop. Errors on [dʒ] are fewer, but occasionally one sees the displacement of [dʒ] by an *affricated* [d], so that "jump" sounds remotely like "dzump." (A plosive sound is said to be *affricated* when it is pronounced with a perceptible fricative release).

In summary, the common sound substitutions of infantile speech are as follows:

[w] or [j]/l	[f]/[θ]
Non-*r*-colored vowel/[ɝ], [ɚ]	[v]/[ð]
[θ]/[s] or [s]/[θ]	[h]/[θ]
[ð]/[z] or [z]/[ð]	[t]/[k]
[l̥]/[s] (lateral lisp)	[d]/[g]
[h]/[s]	[ʔ]/[g], [k], [t], [d],
[θ]/[ʃ]	or other sounds
[ð]/[ʒ]	[w] or [j]/[l]
[s]/[ʃ]	Vowel/[l] (final)
[z]/[ʒ]	[ʃ]/[tʃ]
	[dz]/[dʒ]

There is no firm relationship between the etiology of an articulation disorder and particular phonetic lapses. A given etiology does not always produce the same misarticulations, and, conversely, similar misarticulations can arise from quite different causes. It can be said, however, that the misarticulations described above are those most likely to be found in children whose difficulty springs from an uncomplicated delay in the *maturation* of their phonetic skills. This is not to say that maturational delay is unimportant, or that it can be ignored because the child will outgrow his problem.

Delay in the growth of articulation skills can range from a mild defect to speech that is completely unintelligible. The terms *idiolalia* and *idioglossia* are both used to designate jargon speech. In some cases a child's jargon may be unintelligible because of an extremely limited repertoire of sounds. Alternatively, his speech may contain so many sound substitutions and other errors of the kind described above that it cannot be understood. In such cases one can, by careful phonetic analysis, usually find at least some sound combinations which resemble familiar words. Other jargon talkers employ bizarre and unusual sound substitutions, omissions, or other errors which are quite unlike those of infantile speech. The child's utterance may contain genuine *neologisms* (invented words) used consistently, or it may consist of a kind of phonetic conglomerate with no detectable symbolic function. In either case, some cause other than a simple lag in maturation is likely.

Phonemic Errors Associated with Sensory and Perceptual Deficit

The nature of misarticulations secondary to sensory hearing loss is governed by a number of variables. They depend first on the frequencies at which the individual's threshold is impaired. A *flat audiogram,* in which the loss is approximately the same from 125 Hz to 8,000 Hz, may reduce the child's ability to hear, and therefore learn, any of the sounds of speech. A *high frequency* loss confined to, or greater in, the frequencies lying above 2,000 Hz will have a relatively greater effect on the reception and learning of the fricative, plosive, and affricate sounds than on vowels and diphthongs. The severity of the loss is, of course, of great importance. In addition there are subtle factors, many of them poorly understood, that cannot be deduced from inspection of a routine audiogram, but which nevertheless are critical to the functional efficiency of hearing. Age, intelligence, extent of previous speech learning, and what might be called *phonetic aptitude* are influential variables.

For these and other reasons one must not be too hasty in reaching conclusions about the relationship between auditory acuity and articulation status. Receptive deficits as an etiology will be examined further in Chapter 4; however, we can say generally that a hearing loss present at birth or acquired early in life must be considered one of the significant reasons for misarticulation, and that the patterns of speech are somewhat distinctive for different degrees and kinds of loss.

Phonemic errors in mild hearing loss

By a mild hearing loss, we mean one in which the threshold, while not normal, is still not raised to the point where the child has any significant difficulty in acquiring the ability to talk. The errors in mild hearing loss are primarily on the nonsyllabic fricative, plosive, and affricate sounds. Vowels and other syllabic sounds are little affected because they contain sufficient acoustic energy to bring them above the threshold. Consonants are more difficult to hear and discriminate. Fricative sounds are more vulnerable in this respect than plosives and affricates, again because of differences in acoustic energy.

Actually, the errors in mild hearing loss are much the same as those of infantile speech, which is what one would expect if he accepts the premise that lack of good auditory discrimination is among the major reasons for phonetic delay. Specifically, a child with a mild hearing loss is likely to exhibit [θ]/[s], [ð]/[z], [θ]/[ʃ], [ð]/[ʒ], [s]/[ʃ], [z]/[ʒ], [f]/[θ], [v]/[ð], and similar confusions. Some distortions or inaccurate approximations of the sibilants may be heard, and there may even be a kind of generalized imprecision in articulation. Omission of sounds is not particularly typical.

Phonemic errors of the deaf

Since deafness is defined educationally as a degree of hearing loss so great that the individual has too little hearing to acquire speech (at least without special training), it follows that the associated articulation problems will be severe. Indeed, a failure to develop standard speech sounds is one of the typical signs of deafness in a young child. Among untrained children whose deafness dates from birth (*congenital deafness*) or is acquired shortly thereafter, any attempts at vocalized communication usually consist almost entirely of undifferentiated vowel-like sounds, or of syllables in which the initiating or terminating "consonant" movements are generalized lip and front-tongue adjustments. The signals so produced only remotely resemble familiar speech sounds. Frequently the vowel or vowel-like resonances are conspicuously nasal.

Those deaf children who do acquire some degree of oral speech (and most of them can be taught a great deal) will nevertheless continue to have articulation defects of a kind consistent with the fact that they get few or no auditory cues. The quality of their vowel resonance is almost never accurate enough to make the vowels indistinguishable from those of a normal speaker, although front vowels are often better than back vowels. Consonant articulation is almost certain to be inaccurate, except possibly for the visible sounds, such as [f], [v], [m], [w], and perhaps [θ] and [ð]. Speech sounds ordinarily made with contact between the front of the tongue and the anterior portion of the upper dental arch (*linguapalatal* and *lingua-alveolar* sounds), such as [t], [d], [l], and [n] will usually be better pronounced than *linguavelars* such as [k] [g], and [ŋ], which the deaf child is likely to produce with a fronted position of the tongue. Indeed, all of his *lingual* nonsyllabics are usually made with *lingua-alveolar, linguapalatal,* or *linguadental* positioning.

Both the fricatives and affricates present great difficulties for one who has never heard them. When a deaf child's speech does contain any of these sounds they are usually grossly distorted. A typical pattern is an approximation of [t] for both [s] and [ʃ], so that "see" roughly resembles "tee" and "shoe" sounds something like "too." Equivalents of either [tʃ] and [dʒ] may be dentalized and affricated versions of [t] and [d] ("tsoo" for "chew" and "dzoe" for "Joe").

Voicing or *sonancy* errors are common in the deaf speaker's non-syllabic sounds, the tendency being to add some voicing to what should be voiceless sounds. The duration of the *continuants* (sounds which are not *stop-plosives*) is usually longer than in normal articulation. The degree of force imparted to the *plosives* is typically excessive. When these misarticulations are combined with the prominent nonphonemic defects such as faulty stress, inflection, melody, and vocal quality, the result is typical deaf speech which is easily recognized by anyone familiar with it.

The worsening of articulation in a person whose hearing loss was acquired through injury or disease after he learned to talk is often mentioned. Such deterioration can certainly occur, but it is probably less of a problem than one might infer from some of the comments in the literature. If the hearing loss occurred after articulation was established, say, after the tenth birthday, there may be surprisingly little change in articulation, although it is prudent to apply reasonable measures to conserve speech by teaching the child to make maximum use of nonauditory cues (touch, kinesthesia, vision) for articulation monitoring. At this point in life, *proprioceptive feedback* has become more important in maintaining the fidelity of articulation, and the sense of hearing is not absolutely indispensable. The deterioration of articulation that does occur is largely a general loss of accuracy or "blurring of the outlines" of the sounds in running speech, along with some minimal changes in *prosody*. Vocal quality is usually little affected. Of course, the earlier the onset of deafness, the greater the threat to articulation.

26   Consult O'Neill (216) and Di Carlo (71) for further descriptions of the speech of the hard of hearing and deaf.

Phonemic errors associated with moderate to severe hearing loss

Moderate to severe hearing loss covers the range of auditory disability between mild hearing loss and deafness. Since the range is great, the kind and amount of speech handicap varies considerably.

In general, a moderate to severe loss is sufficiently great to interfere appreciably with language learning and social functioning, and it usually calls for special educational management. The phonemic errors of children with this degree of loss (if congenital, or acquired early) will fit into the patterns described for mild hearing impairments, but will be aggravated in degree. As the severity of the loss approaches deafness, the speech characteristics will naturally become more like those of the deaf.

Retardation in the rate at which phonetic skills are developed is thus more marked than among children with mild hearing loss, but less, of course, than among the deaf. In contrast to mild hearing loss, a moderate to severe loss is likely to cause some misarticulation of the vowels, particularly when the loss of acuity approaches the upper limits of the range. Confusions and misarticulations involving such relatively high energy sounds as [l], [r], [j], [w], [m], [n], and [ŋ] will begin to appear at progressively higher levels of loss; errors on the nonsyllabic sounds will become more nearly like those heard in deaf speakers. Errors in the production of the sibilants and on [f], [v], [θ], and [ð] become more marked, and most of the phonemic confusions characteristic of infantile speech will appear to an aggravated degree. The prosodic elements of speech will also be affected to an extent consistent with the severity of the loss.

Phonemic errors associated with perceptual deficit

Not much can be said with confidence about perceptual deficit except, of course, that it is unquestionably a major source of defective articulation. It may well be that many of the speech errors caused by imperception are not peculiar to it. For instance, the defects characteristic of developmental delay that are thought to be caused by faulty discrimination are possibly more a product of imperception than anything else. It is also interesting to note that brain-injured adults with perceptual defects occasionally talk as though they were in the early stages of speech development.

27   Goldstein (105) describes this phenomenon.

Severe and persistent idiolalia is a recognized symptom of neurological impairment in children, and the concensus of clinical opinion is that this symptom is caused primarily by the perceptual disabilities that are known to exist in the neurologically impaired. Some of these children show a pattern of phonemic errors quite like those of delayed maturation, but they are singularly unable to progress in therapy to the same degree that they may learn in other areas. Perceptual deficit must always be suspected in individuals whose infantile speech leaves traces in their adult years, as is sometimes the case. The phonemic errors of children with imperception resemble, on the whole, those heard in more aggravated cases of sensory hearing disability. Sometimes prosody is like that of the deaf. Marked insensitivity to environmental sound is also a common observation.

28   Mykelbust (207) is a standard reference on these matters.

Phonemic errors associated with structural defects

The misarticulations associated with structural defects of the mouth are difficult to describe systematically because they are so varied, and because they are modified so greatly by functional factors.[1] The *morphogenic* defects of articulation can be a product of (1) inability to channel the breath stream for the production of certain sounds, or (2) difficulties in accomplishing linguapalatal, lingua-alveolar, labiodental, linguadental or bilabial contacts.

Upper arch deformities, such as those associated with clefts of the jaw and dental malocclusions, impair the sibilants particularly because of deviations in the anterior mouth surfaces against which the breath must be channeled for these sounds. The sibilants, labials, labiodentals, and linguadentals are likely to be affected by underbite. In this condition the lower arch is mesial (forward) from its normal position, and this disturbed relationship interferes with positioning of the tongue for post-dental contacts and channeling of the breath stream in the upper arch. The tongue is forced into a position which gives an approximation of [θ] or [ð] for the sibilants. Severe underbite may prevent occlusion of the lips for the labials, which must then be made as labiodentals. [f] and [v] may also be affected. A high narrow upper arch, which is found in many kinds of malocclusion, may interfere with the linguavelar contacts necessary for [k] and [g], and with the linguapalatal or lingua-alveolar contacts for [t], [d], and [l]. Sibilant quality may also be disturbed by a high narrow upper arch. Malposed or missing teeth may create openngs that affect all of the sibilant sounds.

[1] Structurally based defects and the complications inherent in the relationship between structure and function are considered in detail in Chapter 5.

The most common major congenital orofacial defect is cleft palate, a structural deformity that may have serious effects on nearly
all aspects of speech. Functional weakness of the soft palate after
surgery or a palate which is too short to make adequate closure will
cause weakness and underarticulation of all the nonsyllabic sounds
because intraoral breath pressure is insufficient. Wide individual
differences will be found among cleft-palate speakers, but generally
[tʃ], [dʒ], [s], [z], [k], and [g] will be the most defective sounds.
Others that may be involved are the fricatives [f], [v], [θ], and [ð],
and the plosives [t], [d], [p], and [b]. Some authorities report that
the cleft-palate speaker has greatest difficulty with the plosives. A
conspicuous nasal fricative sound caused by nasal air loss often
accompanies the non-syllabic sounds, and undesirable facial movements can sometimes be observed. *Hypernasality* and occasionally
other defects in resonance impair production of all of the voiced
sounds, but are most prominent on the syllabics. One can also find
misarticulations that are not a direct result of the cleft.

29   Westlake and Rutherford (334) give a more detailed description of
cleft-palate speech. Compare their treatment of the subject with that
of Morley (199).

Phonemic errors associated with cultural and environmental factors

Cultural and environmental influences can result in a great
variety of speech conditions, since the forces that can come into
play during the learning period are so numerous. Many of the traits
of *foreign dialect* (sometimes called *barbaralalia*) are nonphonemic,
such as melody, stress, and other prosodic elements. Phonemic defects depend largely on the differences and similarities between
English and the speaker's native language. He may well have
trouble learning sounds which are completely new to him, but
often the English sounds that have some counterpart in his native
language are even more difficult. For instance, sounds from the
r-family are found in many modern languages, but are sufficiently
unlike [r] to make them correct for English speech. The foreign
speaker, however, persists in the use of the *r* with which he is familiar.

30   See Chreist (58) for a full treatment of foreign dialect.

Regional dialect will not be treated here, partly because of space
limitations, but mostly it cannot properly be called defective articulation in most cases. Dialect variations are tolerable for most pur-

poses, unless they are substandard even in the speaker's own dialect region.

31 Wise (338) has an extended description of regional and foreign dialect in his book on applied phonetics, and Carrell and Tiffany (50) have some comments on standards of speech which are relevant to this discussion.

The standards of speech in the child's immediate environment have a profound effect on the way in which he learns to talk. If the speech he hears around him is poor, then his probably will be too, sometimes to the point where he passes the boundary between normal and defective. *Substandard* speech cannot be described here, but see Carrell and Tiffany (50). If a parent, sibling, or playmate has a speech defect he may acquire it too by direct imitation.

Phonemic errors associated with motor deficiencies

These fall generally into two closely related categories: (1) the misarticulations of dysarthria in which disorders of movement are caused by some demonstrable neuropathology, and (2) functional misarticulations, in which there is a definite impairment of motion or coordination without any other evidence of central nervous system pathology.

Much of motor-impaired articulation consists of what we have chosen to call *configurational* and *contextual* defects, such as faulty rhythm in connected speech, but in general the difficulties in producing specific sounds are consistent with the same underlying difficulties in movement. Whenever weakness or a reduction in muscle tone is present, the overall impression is one of imprecise, "mouthed," or "mumbled" articulation in which the movements are not made with sufficient agility. In such cases audibility is reduced, and the speaker may be nasal because of a weakness in the palatopharyngeal complex of muscles. As in nearly all forms of dysarthria, articulation deteriorates as the speed and complexity of the attempted movements increases. In milder cases the term *oral inaccuracy* might be an apt description; in more severe conditions the ability to execute articulation movements may be almost entirely lost (sometimes termed *anarthria*). Phonemic symptoms of this kind may be heard in *bulbar* or *pseudobulbar palsy*. The phonemic features of ataxic speech are much the same, but the loss of fine control also causes disorders of rhythm which are different from those in which there is only weakness.

The articulation symptoms in cerebral palsy are quite distinctive although they vary in severity from mild clumsiness to almost complete disability. Spastic speech is typically slow, labored, and effortful. In athetosis articulation is much the same, but in this form of *dyskinesia* there is more of an explosive, jerky, or irregular quality to the speech movements. If the laryngeal and respiratory musculature are involved, which is possible in both spasticity and athetosis, the coordinated activity of the articulators is further impaired.

32   McDonald and Chance (181) have an extended description of speech defects in cerebral palsy.

No distinctive syndrome can be identified for the functional motor disabilities. Imprecision or clumsiness leading to oral inaccuracy which becomes progressively more uncoordinated in more complex articulation movements is usually prominent in these cases. Simple syllabic movements may be performed relatively well but the blends or consonant clusters are defective. Children with functional disabilities are usually also slower than normal in acquiring phonetic skills. A full description of the acquired *apractic* lapses is given in Chapter 6, but briefly these range from a mild oral inaccuracy or "stumbling" on sounds to the complete inability to execute speech movements. Unusual difficulty in learning neuromuscular patterns for the sounds of speech is thought to be traceable sometimes to apractic-like conditions of developmental origin, presumably a form of central nervous system dysfunction.

33   See Schlesinger (259) for further theoretical and clinical information on apraxia.

Phonemic errors associated with emotional factors

The speech symptoms of abnormal emotional function, like those related to perceptual deficits, often resemble the misarticulations associated with other etiologies. Among children, infantile speech is often emotionally based, reflecting immaturity, insecurity, or some other psychological influence. Infantile speech to which a child regresses after having had normal speech must be regarded as invariably psychogenic. *Dynamic overlay,* or emotional reaction to a disorder of any etiology, may result in its perpetuation, probably to an extent directly proportional to the amount of stress the problem has caused. Cases of a true invented language, where a meaningful jargon with rudimentary linguistic structure serves the child, are always either based on abnormal emotional function or at least have emotional overtones. These invented languages have no distinguishing phonemic features. They consist of bizarre configurations of sound usually mingled with some "words" that remotely resemble those of conventional language. Another form of jargon is heard in the early stages of *primary infantile autism*. Emotional stress may also cause a speaker to make no more than minimal articulation movements.

CONFIGURATIONAL AND CONTEXTUAL DEFECTS

Although phonetic errors are usually classified as sound substitutions, omissions, distortions, and transpositions, it is our hypothesis that certain distinctive disturbances in articulation exist which we have chosen to call *configurational* and *contextual* defects. This hypothesis rests on the premise that these defects represent a kind of dysfunction different from the phonemic errors just described, both in the way they sound and, to a degree, in their etiology. More specifically, *configurational errors* are distinguished by the inability to *sequence* phonetic elements (sound and syllables) into the configurations for words or to *complete* sufficiently large groups of these elements to form words. The latter can be thought of as a limitation in *motor response span*. If the hypothesis is tenable, both are deficiencies in the higher neurophysiological processes that underly articulated speech. *Contextual errors* are the somewhat more familiar disturbances in rate, melody, and stress that appear only in connected speech. Contextual errors also indicate a breakdown in the integrative function of the brain, either in the primary motor effector system or in the higher motor integrative circuitry.

Sequencing elements into a desired whole response is necessary for many kinds of human behavior. In language formulation, verbal symbols must be sequenced so as to conform to the syntactic rules of the language, and one of the signs of disordered language processes in both adults and children is incorrect ordering or transposition of words in propositional speech. A similar sequencing of phonetic elements is necessary for the patterns of normal articulation. Clinically, the "garbling" of phonetic elements within words is often a part of the idiolalia associated with neurological impairment in children, and is also seen in adults with brain damage. Such defects are probably related to the perceptual aspects of higher brain processes in some cases. Children with relatively minor sequencing difficulties can be thought of as suffering from a functional disturbance of the higher processes which is different only in degree from the more aggravated defects associated with neurological impairment.

The omission of sounds is a feature of several kinds of defective articulation. Such errors are common in infantile speech, where pronounciations such as "-ook" for "look," "ba-" for "ball," and "-i-ter" for "sister" will be heard frequently—either with or without other kinds of errors. There is a tendency for these omissions to involve either initial or final phonetic elements of words, although there are exceptions. Mentally retarded children often omit sounds. Omissions may also result from sensory defects in the deaf and hard of hearing, or from perceptual limitations. What some authorities have called deficiencies in *auditory memory span* fit into this context.

The *contextual errors* in which focal or diffuse lesions in the brain prevent normal operation of the primary motor effector system are readily understandable. Defects in rate, rhythm, and stress are prominent in all forms of cerebral palsy. The spastic individual cannot, because of his underlying motor handicap, maintain normal speech rhythms. His articulation is reduced in rate, his pitch changes are not appropriate to intellectual and emotional meanings, and the loss of muscular control prevents him from carrying out the changes in stress which are necessary to normal speech. In athetosis, rate, melody, and stress are all impaired, but the adjectives, *jerky, irregular,* and *explosive,* are most descriptive, in contrast to the slow, labored, effortful articulation of the spastic. Ataxic speech is difficult to describe verbally. There is usually an over-all flaccidity or weakness of movement which is sometimes described as sounding as if the speaker "had a hot potato in his mouth." "Scanning" or monotonous articulation is found in cerebellar ataxia. This refers to the absence of the fine nuances of rate, melody, and stress—normally mediated by the cerebellar system—which convey intellectual and emotional meaning. Contextual errors in bulbar and pseudobulbar palsy occur only insofar as weakness of motion interferes with the rhythm of articulation. When the higher integrative circuits are impaired, the speaker does not lose the ability to execute the individual components of the total pattern of movement, but he cannot successfully combine these movements into normal connected speech, so that "Methodist Episcopal" becomes something such as "Methus piscul."

FUNCTIONAL DISORDERS OF ARTICULATION, TO WHICH THE TERM *dyslalia* is applied, are generally defined as those in which articulation functioning is abnormal in an individual who is presumed to have no structural or physiological deficit to which his speech defect can be attributed. Categorizing on the basis of the *predominating etiology,* functional defects constitute approximately 75 per cent of all disorders of articulation. Furthermore functional influences arising *from* the speech defect complicate nearly every case.

The functional causes of articulation disorders will be considered here under the following headings: (1) *psychosocial* factors; (2) deficiencies or defects of *intelligence;* (3) *receptive deficits* of a sensory and perceptual nature, and (4) *delayed maturation.* It is

3

functional factors: psychosocial influences

evident that these categories are by no means mutually exclusive.

The term *psychosocial* is used in this context to refer to (1) *habit strength,* insofar as it contributes to the persistence of defective articulation; (2) the *environmental influences* that shape a child's speech; and (3) the complex *psychodynamic* forces that affect an individual's personality structure and hence his social behavior, including communication.

HABIT STRENGTH

The importance of habits in human motor behavior is self-evident. The ability to form habits enables us to carry out literally hundreds of necessary activities without having to pay conscious attention to what we are doing. But the automaticity which make habits so useful is a disadvantage in that, once fixed at the automatic level, wrong patterns of response persist unless there is some form of intervention. Once established, then, defective articulation continues until special measures are taken to break the old habits and form new ones. The original cause of the speech defect is, in a sense, irrelevant; even if it is removed the defect remains because habit maintains it.

The principles governing all motor habits are the same, but there are some features of the habits of articulation that are distinctive and difficult to deal with. In some respects they have a higher degree of automaticity than many other motor habits. When a child learns to write, for instance, he is very aware of the model he is trying to imitate, and when he tries to form the letters he pays close attention to the movements of his hand and arm. He continues this deliberate self-monitoring until the habits are established. In learning to speak, however, he pays little or no conscious attention to either the model or the movements he makes to imitate it. Patterns of movement have been established during the babbling and vocal play periods; input-output loops for imitating speech have already been established and operate at a far lower level of consciousness than those used in the movements for writing, putting on one's cap, or turning a door knob. Even when a child's attention is directed to the sound of a word he is being taught or has mispronounced, the interval of conscious listening is very brief. The mother who gives her child good early teaching and thus prevents defective articulation has changed the picture, of course, by bringing the speech learning process to a higher level of consciousness.

Some aspects of motor speech learning are more like walking than writing. Before a child takes his first step he has already developed a readiness for walking: posture, balance, reciprocal leg motion, and so on. Some preparation is necessary for all motor responses, of course, but not to the highly specialized degree found in walking and talking. Articulation is also more difficult to monitor than most motor habits. If a child makes a wrong walking movement, he falls down; if he forms a letter incorrectly in writing, he has the mistake there before his eyes; if he does not turn the knob correctly, the door will not open. If he misarticulates a word, no such readily perceptible consequence follows—particularly if his incorrect response gets him what he wants or is reinforced in some other way.

As a result of all these factors, the articulation responses a child first learns become firmly fixed, whether they lead to speech that is conspicuously deviant or not. The child's primary goal is to communicate, and whatever behavior is rewarded by successful communication becomes habituated quickly. Because his attention is centered on what he is saying, not on his manner of speaking, there is little reason why these habits should not persist, barring outside intervention. The longer an incorrect habit is practiced, the more firmly it becomes entrenched. Consequently there are probably few if any cases of established defective speech in which habit strength does not operate independently of the original cause.

34   Compare what is said here about habit strength with the comments of Van Riper (318) on the same subject.

ENVIRONMENTAL INFLUENCES

The standards of speech in a child's environment are obviously a major factor in determining his own way of talking. Whatever language is spoken in his environment will be the one he learns, and his speech will also mirror the particular dialect of those around him. If he is exposed to substandard or defective speech at home or in the neighborhood during the first months and years of his life, he is almost certain to use it himself. Neither a later change of environment nor the most extensive tutoring is likely to eradicate his speech origins entirely. Environmental influences must be considered among the more common functional factors in defective articulation.

Foreign Language Influences

Among children foreign dialect problems are mostly confined to a limited number of areas. One must nevertheless be aware that the use of a foreign language in the home, dialect traits in one or both parents or in the community, or some other special circumstance—for instance, a child having spent his early years in another country—may impair his mastery of English speech. Foreign language influences become less important as the child grows older and widens his circle of acquaintances, and the more prominent signs of foreign dialect usually clear up rapidly in the course of early school experiences. If they do not, speech improvement is in order. It is only when speech and language have become thoroughly habituated that a shift to a second language creates serious problems.

There are differences of opinion on the possible hazards of *bilingualism*. Some feel that there is considerable risk in exposing an immature child to two languages during his speech learning period, partly because of the added difficulty he will experience in acquiring two expressive vocabularies, and partly because of the stress that this potentially confusing language environment may create. Others think that bilingualism *per se* is not a major cause of articulation or language problems. There is no convincing evidence in either direction, and probably each case should be judged individually.

35   Berry and Eisenson (26) discuss bilingualism in some detail and summarize a number of the research studies on the topic.

An adult learning a second language is certain to encounter problems which, for economic and social reasons, he may need very bady to solve. Some of his phonemic errors and his difficulties with prosody were touched on earlier, but many teachers who have worked with foreign students believe that the focus of instruction should be on language, rather than pronounciation. They feel that articulation is secondary, and that many of the speech errors are corrected most easily after the individual has learned to think in his new language. In any case, habit strength must be overcome in shifting to a second language. *Regional dialect,* which at the worst

36   See Chreist (58) for an excellent treatment of the whole subject of foreign dialect.

causes only minor defects of articulation, has the same general etiology as foreign dialect, and is similarly maintained by habit strength.

Speech Models

The speech models that other people provide a child during the formative years of his life have the greatest possible influence on his speech. First in importance are the speech standards of the home which the parents unconsciously impose on him; his own way of talking will reflect the pronunciation, melody, and even vocal quality he hears in the adults who care for him or to whom he is most often exposed. The child has a normal tendency to identify with another figure, a tendency which leads him to emulate unconsciously the mannerisms, personality traits, and behavior traits, including speech, of the person he wishes to be like. "He talks just like his father" is a common observation which is easy to explain.

Whether or not a child acquired his defective speech solely by imitating another child or an adult is occasionally an important diagnostic question and a matter of great concern to the parents. Certainly defective speech in a brother, sister, playmate, or parent can have an unfavorable effect, but one should not be too ready to accept this explanation for a child's articulation disorder. It is common, when an older brother or sister has a speech problem, for the parents to fear that it will cause a similar defect in the younger child. This can happen, but one must remember that the child hears these unsuitable models only a fraction of the time. Ordinarily he is also exposed to other and better speech models which should counteract the poor models unless some force other than simple imitation is at work.

Many times the younger child's errors are only a normal stage in development, even though they mirror the articulation defect of an older child. With siblings, it is always possible that, rather than imitation, the same etiology is responsible for similar articulation problems in the two children. Although defective speech can be acquired by imitation, one should explore other possible causes thoroughly.

The notion that parental baby talk is one of the main causes of infantile speech seems to have become part of our folklore. It is possible that a two-year-old who constantly hears himself addressed as "muvver's pwecious" might fall into the practice of saying words the same way. The parent's failure to provide a good speech model or proper home teaching is always a potential source of trouble. In most cases, however, the more important influence is the emotional climate which causes the parents to use baby talk excessively, that is, their tendency to foster the child's social and emotional immaturity.

Twins, or other children who have an unusually close relationship, sometimes develop an invented language. Such a language usually contains words that are similar to their conventional counterparts, along with *neologisms,* which are truly invented words serving a linguistic function. Invented languages may contain extensive vocabularies, have a rudimentary grammar and syntax, and be spoken fluently by those who are privy to its secrets. It will be lingo to others, however, although Mother or an older sibling may learn to understand it fairly well. Sometimes one twin will speak English too and act as interpreter.

Up to a point these invented languages develop in perfectly lawful ways. The vocalizations of one child become associated with a meaning, and the chance pattern of sound is reinforced by a response from the other child. The round object that bounces can just as easily become "goop" as "ball" if circumstances are right— and they may be with twins who are constantly together and developing simultaneously. A similar process occurs when an adult adopts a child's unsuccessful efforts to say words; this is how household words arise, so that grandfather becomes "Bops" and grandmother something else unique.

Although nearly universal to some degree in twins and not unusual in other children, invented words normally disappear as soon as the children pass beyond the toddling stage. Certainly an invented language should be nearly forgotten by late preschool years, although a few words may remain. When this does not happen one may suspect either that the parents' teaching methods were very poor or that there is some emotional abnormality in the situation. In aggravated cases the latter is more likely. The degree of emotional interdependence which would cause two children to cling to this mode of communication is not normal and may, in severe cases, have reached the proportions of a morbid *symbiotic* relationship. When an adult, perhaps the mother, is involved in the conspiracy, abnormal emotionality becomes a virtual certainty.

The management of this problem calls for intelligent preventive teaching by the parents, possibly speech help outside the home at an appropriate time, perhaps a degree of physical separation (separate nursery schools, for instance), or any other measures which will discourage the reinforcement of the invented language. When emotional factors are considered significant, and this is almost always the case, treatment should focus on them. The true invented language, however, must be differentiated from the jargon speech of the retarded, neurologically impaired, autistic, and other kinds of children to be discussed in later sections.

Environmental Deprivation

If a child were raised in virtual isolation, as occasionally happens, he would acquire no more speech than meaningless undifferentiated vocalizations and emotional interjections, and perhaps not many of these. Similarly, a lack of adequate stimulation from the environment may be a cause of defective articulation. Except in extraordinary circumstances, most children hear speech, although the kind and amount vary widely. Sometimes the family group is simply not talkative, or there are no siblings or playmates. Circumstances that reduce stimulation are not in the least unusual. To mention a few examples, children with normal hearing may be born to speechless deaf parents; working mothers sometimes cannot avoid leaving their children with a minimum of adult care; prolonged illness can reduce speech stimulation (and introduce other factors as well); and so on. A generally impoverished environment—economically, socially, or culturally—can also have far-reaching effects on all aspects of a child's development. One must remember that understimulation or environmental deprivation cannot possibly exist without introducing at least some degree of emotional deprivation, so that it should never be viewed narrowly as simply a lack of opportunity to learn speech.

Another cause of defective articulation is the failure of the parents to encourage and guide the child's early speech development. He may retain infantilisms or other misarticulations because he is neither made aware of them nor given the kind of speech help parents normally should provide. In such cases defective articulation is reinforced because it serves the child's need perfectly well; once established these errors become increasingly difficult to eradicate as time passes. Parents who neglect to give speech help may simply be uninformed, but here again one should look closely for feelings and attitudes which may keep the parents from playing their normal roles in stimulating the child's development.

> 37   There are a number of references which elaborate on the theory and method of speech stimulation for developing children. Compare, for instance, Van Riper (319) and Jones (149).

PSYCHO-DYNAMIC FACTORS

Complex psychological forces often impair communication, and they can do so in a variety of ways. Psychological influences can cause a child to cling to infantile articulation and they can cause him to be socially maladjusted in some way that is reflected in his speech. Some children regress from normal to infantile speech for emotional reasons. Emotional and personality problems, in fact, can cause abnormality in all aspects of the speech of older children and adults. When penalties of one kind or another have made speech a significant source of stress and anxiety, an individual may cling to his defect for unconscious satisfaction of his emotional needs and reject help. The psychological forces that cause defective speech are so complex that we can do no more than sketch them briefly.

One important cause of defective speech is unsatisfactory *personality structure*. That talking reveals traits of personality is, of course, a matter of common knowledge, but the relationship between the two is so critical for understanding certain kinds of defective speech that some elaboration of underlying theory is called for. As psychologists use the term, *personality* means the aggregate of an individual's traits and ways of behaving which, by reason of their unique organization, account for the way he adjusts to his environment, and make him "the kind of person he is." There are many theories to explain personality development and the influences that are most important in determining personality structure but these need not concern us here.

38   If the reader is unfamiliar with the theories of personality he should consult one of the basic texts in general psychology, such as Sanford (252) or Hilgard (124).

We are greatly concerned, however, with the fact that speech is a form of social behavior which emerges in the child only if his personality structure develops in such a way that he comes to relate normally to his environment. A child's first talking and the subsequent expansion and elaboration of verbal behavior are evidence of normal social and emotional growth, that is, he is developing into the kind of socialized being who interacts with others through talking, as well as in other ways.

It follows, then, that abnormalities in communication may come about whenever an adverse influence prevents a child from achieving the normal amount and quality of *interpersonal relatedness* he should have to function successfully. Changes in established communicative behavior can occur later if traumatic forces disturb an individual so seriously that he can no longer maintain a normal adjustment to his social environment. In a developing child a first communication disorder related to emotional abnormalty may be a deficiency in the *quantity* of speech. In such cases, the child may have little or no speech because he has not established the kind of interpersonal relationships out of which talking grows. He may also be delayed *qualitatively,* in which case his phonetic skills are retarded because he has no need for, or does not want, the kind of relationships he can establish only by talking intelligibly. In this event, defective articulation will be a prominent feature of his problem.

It should be clear, then, that one must bring to bear all that is known about normal and deviant personality growth in order to understand some of the functional disorders of articulation. Although personality structure depends partly on innate factors, one must look particularly for influences in the social and physical environment which have shaped the child's ways of thinking and feeling in such a way that his relating behavior is incompatible with normal communication.

Infantile speech is one of the conditions often related to emotional factors. Sometimes the mechanisms of such social and emotional immaturity appear rather uncomplicated, at least on the surface, but in many cases they are complex and difficult to deal with. Occasionally the child has simply not had the kind of social experience that encourages the process of growing up. He may, for instance, have had few playmates at home or in the neighborhood. Nursery schools or preschool speech stimulation groups which emphasize social interaction are excellent under these circumstances.

Parenthetically, parents often worry about whether a child with marked infantile speech should start school at the regular age or be held out until his speech has been corrected. If the child is otherwise ready, the social experiences of kindergarten or first grade are exactly what he needs.

Immaturity in development is more often a product of the *kind* of relationship the child has to the world around him than a lack of social experiences. The child may have been kept immature by the adults around him. One or both parents may have fostered his dependency in order to satisfy emotional needs of their own, or, for one reason or another, the child himself may need to remain dependent. Both forces may be at work, since one tends to generate the other. A dependency relationship may gratify a parent's emotional needs in many ways. For example, anything that induces anxiety in a parent may cause him, through a mechanism sometimes called *displacement,* to focus his feelings on the child. Thus, if a mother's security is threatened by marital discord or some other circumstance, she may try to make the child more dependent on her.

Unconscious feelings of rejection toward a handicapped child, combined with a sense of guilt, can lead to a *reaction formation* that ends in overprotection. This psychological mechanism allows the parent to deny feelings of rejection that he is unable to recognize or face. *Ambivalent* attitudes—mixed or alternating feelings of love and hate—are perfectly normal reactions for a parent to have toward any child, but a severely handicapped child may arouse these feelings much more intensely. While the child's condition brings into play strong maternal and paternal protective instincts, the existence of the defective child is, at the same time, an unconscious *ego threat* to the parent. Unrecognized feelings of *hostility* become a part of the total reaction. *Guilt* is generated by these unresolved conflicts. These illustrations are quite inadequate for any deep understanding of the range of psychological problems that can affect articulation, but they may at least suggest directions in the identification of functional causes of articulation disorders.

For normal social and emotional growth the child needs a stable, secure, stimulating, and accepting environment in which he experiences pleasant and rewarding interpersonal relationships which reinforce communication. An infant's most important relationship is with his mother and this continues to be true for a long period of time. Disturbances in this relationship are frequently found among children with marked immaturity or some form of maladaptive behavior. A problem of this kind is often associated with the physical separation of the mother and child caused by illness of either one, a broken home, or any one of a large number of contingencies. Perhaps of even greater significance is the emotional isolation a child suffers from a cold, rigid, rejecting, or unstable mother.

As time passes the mother-child relationship continues to be important, but other relationships emerge to influence the child's social and emotional development. The process of *identification*—the boy with his father and girl with her mother—plays a significant part in the process of maturation. Eventually the need to relate to other children comes to the fore as the child's activities are expanded to the yard, the playground, and later the school. Many acute problems can arise at this point, particularly for handicapped children, if satisfying, enjoyable relationships cannot be established with peers. At this age social growth is rapid, and an interruption of the process can seriously damage the child's emotional health. Within the family, *sibling rivalry* can generate strong feelings and aberrant behavior, sometimes regressive, as in a return to infantile speech, when the child feels threatened by a brother or sister.

Other things which threaten the stability and security of the child's environment can have an adverse effect, such as frequent changes in residence or shifts from one school to another. Financial difficulties or other family crises can easily provoke emotional conflicts. Marital discord is a particularly likely source of insecurity because of the interacting feelings of those involved, and because the child is always an involuntary participant. Poor methods of discipline, too rigid, too permissive, unreasonable, or inconsistent, are also a frequent cause of instability. In short, any stress in the physical or social environment can impair a child's emotional growth and development.

Infantile speech is by no means the only kind of articulation problem that can stem from emotional origins. As suggested earlier, invented languages are often associated with abnormal emotionality. The neologisms that form these languages may have been acquired by perfectly orderly learning processes, but if they continue to be used for communication, something more than learning is in the picture. Twins who do not spontaneously give up most of their jargon by school age are not relating normally to people other than themselves. A similar kind of unhealthy association is always suspect if a parent and child, or a child and anyone else, use a mode of communication which only they can understand. An understanding of the child's failure to acquire normal speech articulation will depend on an understanding of the psychodynamic reasons for the morbid relationship—and training cannot be successful until these reasons have been dealt with.

Emotional disturbances can also cause *regression* from normal speech to infantile speech, or some other kind of deterioration. The neurotic mechanisms which cause a child to revert to infantile behavior are basically the same as those which cause another child to remain immature, except that they become effective after social and emotional growth has been relatively normal for a time. Thus, there are many possible causes for regressive behavior, although sibling rivalry and other family-centered problems show up often. Improvement is often dramatic in such cases if the cause is dealt with. One child encountered by the writer returned from severe infantile speech to normal articulation within two weeks after his father returned from military service.

Deterioration of articulation is an interesting phenomenon observed in both children and adults. Under stressful circumstances an individual's speech may become slurred, inaccurate, irregular, or otherwise abnormal, to the point where it is unintelligible. Emotional stress is in part responsible for the fact that nearly all children or adults with an articulation disorder talk much worse under pressure than when relaxed and unhurried. There is a curious tendency for vocal quality to become hypernasal, or for nasality to become aggravated. Deviations such as cluttering, oral inaccuracy, and weak or inaudible speech are related more often to emotional stress than to any other factor in physically normal speakers. A ready breakdown of speech under the stresses and strains of everyday life may be considered one of the signs of a neurotic individual.

39   The literature on emotional problems is most extensive, but one general reference that would be relevant to the preceeding discussion is Kessler (156).

Thus far only the effect of outside forces has been considered. Constitutional or inborn factors may also predispose toward conditions of which defective speech is an element. It is generally postulated that such constitutional factors do exist, although they cannot usually be identified with confidence. Nevertheless the case history is strongly suggestive if it contains instability or defect in the family line—neurotic behavior, psychosis, mental deficiency, and so on—even though such data are inconclusive.

In this connection, we should note the *autistic* child, or one who suffers from what is sometimes called *primary infantile autism*. Signs of this syndrome appear sufficiently early in life, at least in some cases, to support the view that the condition is inborn. In general autistic behavior is self-oriented or self-centered. The central feature of the syndrome is the child's failure (or inability) to form appropriate interpersonal relationships. The autistic child, although aware of the people around him, will not interact on a "person to person" level. One of the early signs is a failure to exhibit rudimentary social and relating behavior. For instance, mothers describe these infants as "just feeling different" when held for feeding. They distinctly are not cuddly babies, will not reach to be picked up when they grow a bit older, and in many other similar respects do not react to people in the expected way.

After infancy, lack of communication may be the most observable peculiarity in autistic children, and it is for this reason that so many of them are brought to a speech clinic when their parents become concerned. The typical autistic child usually passes normally through a babbling period, except that he does not babble "socially," and later he does not show *echolalic* or word-imitating behavior like that of a normal child. Vocal play may be generous in amount and culminate in a jargon utterance, but the vocal play is solitary, self-oriented, and not used with any evidence of intent to relate interpersonally with others. Although autistic children are notably late in developing language, most of them do eventually acquire speech. When they do, however, the language content and structure are still not communicative in the ordinary sense, but remain internally oriented. Although it is an incidental part of the total problem, the autistic child's speech may be jargon or even nothing more than undifferentiated vocalization for a protracted period. Most writers report discouraging results in their attempts to work with these children.

40   Kanner (151) is considered a standard reference on primary infantile autism.

Two functional disorders that are more clinical curiosities than anything else for the speech pathologist are the *Gilles de la Tou-*

rette and *cri-du-chat syndromes.* In the first, the child's utterance consists of grunt-like undifferentiated vocalization, barking-like noises, and profanity. It is believed to be psychogenic by most psychiatrists, although abnormal neurological findings have been reported in some cases. The *cri-du-chat* ("cry of the cat") *syndrome* is characterized by the child's use of mewing sounds. Should either of these be encountered, psychiatric referral is indicated.

Finally, *dynamic overlay,* or emotional reactions that are caused by defective speech, must be considered since at times these secondary psychological forces play an important part in maintaining defective articulation. One complication is the development of negative feelings and attitudes toward communication, or toward efforts at speech improvement. It is easy to understand why a child whose talking has been strongly penalized should react defensively either by refusing to talk or by resisting any invasion of his speech privacy. Embarrassing, tactless, or unpleasant criticism of articulation errors may provoke such withdrawal behavior, although anything else that makes communication a source of stress can have the same effect. Speech correctionists should be sensitive to the fact that prolonged training, particularly if it is unsuccessful, is quite likely to induce negativism. Indeed, some feelings of this sort should be anticipated with every case at the start.

41   Van Riper (318) has some suggestions for dealing with negativism.

Secondary gain or *neurotic profit* are familiar concomitants of articulation disorders. A speech defect can serve unconsciously to gain attention, control environment, or relieve guilt. It may seem curious that a child or adult should seek attention in such a socially undesirable way as speaking defectively, yet this occurs, and not uncommonly, just as a child may misbehave in order to command attention he thinks he cannot get otherwise. Defective articulation is used to control people by causing anxiety and concern in those against whom it is directed. It may also be used, like stuttering, to avoid situations and responsibilities the speaker does not wish to face. One cleft-palate speaker known to the author, for instance, cannot wear a speech prosthesis which gives him nearly normal speech because, he complains, "It makes my jaw hurt!" Beyond question the real reason is that he can excuse his lack of success in the profession for which he was educated on grounds of his defective articulation. His guilt feelings are thus reduced. Secondary gain is a powerful negative influence that must often be faced in the training program.

One should never lose sight of the effect that a speech defect—even a "mild" one—may have on social and emotional adjustment. Differences of any sort can be very hard to bear. Because defective speech is a difference that is socially conspicuous, it can have a particularly damaging effect on emotional health. The child who cannot talk, or who cannot make himself understood, suffers a frustration that may have serious emotional consequences which can color his entire life.

THE FUNCTIONAL FACTORS TO BE DISCUSSED IN THE PRESENT CHAPTER embrace a variety of conditions which are of great etiologic significance in disorders of articulation. The first, deficiencies or defects in *intelligence,* produce a number of learning disabilities which impair speech and language. *Receptive deficit,* perhaps the most common single cause of articulation disorders, damages the function of those sensory and perceptual input processes that mediate speech learning. *Delayed maturation* causes the developmental disorders of articulation and involves several aspects of physical and psychological growth. All are interrelated. Remember that although these factors can impair articulation functioning, they are sometimes caused by physiological or organic conditions.

functional factors: intelligence;
receptive deficit;
delayed maturation

4

DEFICIENCIES AND DEFECTS OF INTELLIGENCE

Speech is generally said to be a form of learned behavior. To be entirely accurate, it is not wholly learned since some components of the total speech responses are unlearned behavior acquired through maturation. Nevertheless, learning problems associated with defects and deficiencies in intelligence are a major cause of impaired communication. We will have to broaden our discussion to include language learning since the acquisition of verbal symbols and learning to articulate them are not wholly separable processes.

Articulation disorders are much more frequent among mentally retarded than among normal children. Furthermore, the severity of the articulation defects increases with the degree of retardation. For instance, Burt (41) found that the incidence of defective articulation was 14 per cent in a group of school children with IQ's from 70 to 85 and nearly 25 per cent in those with IQ's from 50 to 70. He also found "severe" disorders in 5 and 13 per cent of the two groups respectively. Other studies have reported similar findings, and in some cases the reported frequency of speech defect in the mentally retarded population was even higher.

42   Several such studies are summarized by Matthews (185).

What exactly is meant by intelligence? Psychologists find it difficult to agree on a definition of the term, but for our purposes a person behaves "intelligently," in the broadest sense, if he is able to solve problems through perceptual, cognitive, and verbal processes, and if he can perform certain tasks involving learning.

But, as Hebb (119) has pointed out, the term *intelligence* can be used in two different senses, and at any given time one must understand which meaning he has in mind. What Hebb calls *Intelligence A* is the individual's innate potential: that level of performance of which he would be capable under the most favorable circumstances. *Intelligence B,* on the other hand, is his average level of performance at a given time. The latter is measured by intelligence tests or estimated from some other observation of his behavior. Intelligence A can be inferred from Intelligence B, but one must give careful consideration to those variables that can cause discrepancies between the two. It cannot be assumed that the two are always the same.

It follows, then, that the terms *mental retardation* and *mental deficiency* should be defined with care. The professional literature is confusing because it often fails to do so. *Mental retardation* is frequently used as a general term for any intellectual disability without recognizing the value of a separate meaning for the term *mental deficiency*. A child should be thought of as *mentally deficient* if his innate potential is limited either by heredity *(endogenous* or *familial* mental deficiency), or by some *exogenous* cause (pre- or postnatal brain damage, for instance). Mental deficiency is, then, a limitation of Intelligence A.

By *mentally retarded* one means that a child's measured intelligence is below the expected level for his age; this is Intelligence B. The degree of retardation depends on how far below the average he falls. If performance is less than potential, we say the child is *functionally retarded* to that extent and the condition is, at least in theory, reversible. Functional retardation can be the result of emotional disturbance, deprivation, sensory or perceptual deficit, insufficient motivation and the like. Moreover, defective speech and language can be a prime cause of functional retardation.

There are some further facts about intelligence in relation to speech that have a practical bearing on communication problems. The tasks selected for intelligence testing are of two basic kinds: *verbal,* or problems requiring language for their solution, and *nonverbal,* or *performance* items, which do not. The assumption is that intellectual functioning has two components, each of which is best measured by a particular kind of task. Some tests, particularly those for preschool children, are made up exclusively of performance items; other tests may contain only verbal tasks. Tests such as the Stanford Binet include both verbal and nonverbal items, and the individual's score is a composite of his ability in these two areas. Still other tests, such as the Wechsler scale, can be scored for *verbal intelligence, nonverbal intelligence,* or both combined (generally referred to as *full scale*).

Intelligence tests can be used for either *classification* or *diagnosis,* which are not quite the same things. When a test is employed for classification, the results are usually expressed in terms of *mental age* or *intelligence quotient* (IQ). A child is said to have a mental age of four years if he passes the test items that have been standardized for average four-year-olds; his intelligence quotient is calculated by dividing mental age by chronological age and multiplying the result by 100 to remove the decimal. Thus, if mental and chronological age are exactly the same the IQ will be 100 and the subject is "average" or "normal." A test score, however, tells us nothing about *why* an individual falls below the normal range, except possibly where separate verbal and nonverbal IQ's are calculated.

A test is used diagnostically when the examiner analyzes the *kinds* of tasks that are failed (memory, reasoning, visuomotor performance, and so on), and the *way* in which the subject performed. The psychologist will also evaluate the subject's reaction to the examiner and to the test situation, the manner in which he worked, his motivation, and other *qualitative* aspects of his behavior.

Classifying a child as "dull normal" or "borderline" on the basis of IQ tells us something about his over-all ability, but it does not tell us how to improve his level of function. For this purpose one needs information about the exact nature of the child's intellectual assets and liabilities, and the manner in which he fails. We cannot make a confident generalization that retarded children are poor prospects for speech and language improvement, since most of the studies on the relationship between mental retardation and communication disorders show only that such children fall below normal when they are *classified* on the basis of mental age or IQ. Speech pathologists are beginning to realize that *diagnostic* appraisal can uncover areas of deficit that can be improved by training, or circumvented by a judicious choice of teaching methods.

Children with language disabilities, of course, do poorly on verbal items, as do many children with articulation disorders. It is sometimes said, therefore, that verbal tests of intelligence are unsuitable for appraisal of these children, and that judgments about their intellectual capacity should be based on performance items, which are "fairer" because they do not penalize language deficiencies. This is not entirely correct. The child's responses to nonverbal items supply a great deal of information about his intellectual function in nonverbal areas, but because the child does have language problems, a test of his verbal abilities is also an indispensable part of any total assessment.

A comprehensive diagnostic test might, for instance, enable the psychologist to say that the child shows evidence of generalized mental deficiency which makes the prognosis for training poor. On the other hand, the results might also suggest that one kind of intellectual ability is better than his apparent verbal intelligence; qualitative analysis might reveal *defects* in function rather than generalized deficiency. A distinction must be made between tests of nonverbal intelligence and those that do not require language for their administration. The examiner can often use gesture, pantomime, or demonstration so that the child's lack of verbal understanding or other receptive deficit will not be a cause for failure.

What does it mean when a child is found to be retarded in verbal intelligence? A point sometimes overlooked in this connection is that anyone with disabilities in language function is *per se* retarded in verbal intelligence insofar as this is inferred from his ability to use language. But it is here that the distinction between Intelligence A and Intelligence B becomes important. Is the *measured* verbal intelligence the same as the *innate potential,* or is the retardation functional? And is retardation due to a specific defect of some kind, or is there, instead, a generalized deficiency in all aspects of verbal intelligence?

These questions can be very hard to answer. If language capacity appears to be *nil,* there is at least a faint ray of hope if nonverbal intelligence proves to be relatively better. The psychological appraisal must utilize whatever cues can be found in a thorough and perceptive analysis of the test results. Unless the child shows unmistakable signs of severe irreversible mental deficiency, it may be that a true appraisal cannot be made until after he has been given *diagnostic teaching* for an adequate length of time. Two other points should be made in this connection. First, even if a child must be classified as mentally deficient and can never become fully normal, there is no defense for not helping him realize his maximum potential. Second, his level of achievement must be considered in relation to his chronological age, since growth may enhance readiness to learn, and the child who is not educable at four years of age may become so when he is older.

It would not be accurate to say that all intelligence tests are designed exclusively as classifying instruments since all of them permit the examiner to make qualitative observations. Nevertheless, as a group they are not designed specifically to break down diagnostically the way in which language processes are impaired. Some advances have been made, however, in the direction of tests that better suit the needs of speech and language clinics. The Illinois Test of Psycholinguistic Abilities devised by McCarthy and Kirk (177), although only indirectly a measure of verbal intelligence, offers a promising approach to the identification of defects in function.

There are many kinds of defective articulation heard in mentally retarded children, probably because there are so many different disabilities that may be involved. Those with borderline intelligence or in the higher ranges of the defective group tend to have infantile speech and are slow in developing phonetic skills. At lower levels there are more phonemic and configurational errors, and, at very low levels, speech is jargon-like and contains bizarre and unusual phonetic lapses. Omission of sounds and incomplete word patterns are prominent. *Oral inaccuracy* is typical, consistent with the poor motor coordination and flaccidity of many of these children.

Inability to learn and use the sounds of speech, however, is not always present in the retarded—a fact that has some implications for their education. Many retarded children, including even those with quite low measured intelligence, have excellent articulation insofar as they have expressive vocabularies. Those who show echolalia— and they are common—may imitate perfectly the words they hear; their difficulties lie in the area of conceptualization and the formulation of propositional speech. Not a great deal of intelligence is needed to learn the phonetic elements of speech, since many normal children of no more than two or two and a half years of age master the sounds of speech. Consequently, mental retardation cannot be considered a complete barrier to intelligible speech.

RECEPTIVE DEFICIT

We mentioned earlier that adequate receptive processes are indispensable to speech and language learning. Obviously, then, receptive deficits are a prime cause of articulation disorders. The discussion that follows will center around two closely related aspects of the receptive processes: (1) *sensory* channels, which carry information about speech to the brain, and (2) *perceptual* functions, through which sensory data are integrated, organized, and recognized.

Sensory Defects

Audition

The sense of hearing must be normal to provide optimum conditions for learning speech, and any reduction in auditory sensitivity can be expected to interfere with the acquisition of phonetic skills to a degree consistent with the amount and kind of hearing loss. Normal hearing has been operationally defined through extensive study of individuals presumed to have normal hearing. The results of these studies have been incorporated in a scale of test values which can be used clinically for the measurement of hearing. Currently. the ISO or International Standards Organization scale has quasi-official status, having largely replaced the older ASA or American Standards Association scale. The sound energies required to make pure tones of certain frequencies just audible to the normal ear are incorporated in the scale, which thus defines the *average lower threshold* of hearing. If hearing is less sensitive than normal, the threshold is raised, and a hearing loss exists. The amount of loss is usually measured in *decibels* (abbreviated dB), a unit that expresses the amount of energy that must be added to the normal threshold intensity to make the sound audible to the person being tested. For measurement purposes the average threshold is assigned a value of 0 dB. If the test tone must be increased 20 dB from this point in order to be audible to the subject, he is said to have a 20 dB hearing loss. The threshold for each test frequency is then recorded on a graph called an *audiogram*. There are, of course, many special problems and techniques in the measurement of hearing, particularly in children.

> 43   Readers who have no orientation in audiology should consult one of the standard references, such as Newby (213) or Davis and Silverman (68).

Speech reception is a complex process which depends on many factors other than the simple sensitivity of the auditory system to sound. Consequently, a routine pure-tone audiogram does not give complete information about an individual's ability to hear the details of speech. In general, however, for optimum articulation learning, the child should have a normal threshold for all frequencies between approximately 100 and 8,000 Hz. Any loss within this range can impair his ability to make the necessary discriminations between similar speech sounds. Speech reception will not be seriously impaired, so far as the understanding of words is concerned, if hearing is normal at 500, 1,000, and 2,000 Hz—the *speech frequencies*—since a major proportion of the energy in the frequencies needed to identify the sounds falls within these limits. Fine discrimination, however, is not fully efficient unless auditory acuity is good over the wider range. One may have a hearing loss up to 40 dB and meet the criteria of *social adequacy,* but even a minimal rise in the threshold can interfere with articulation learning.

A common case in clinical diagnosis is the child who is tested in his late preschool or early school years and proves to have normal hearing, but who has a history of middle-ear disease or one which is presumptive of it. Medical treatment or other factors which improved the child's health may have conserved his hearing, but he may still have been suffering some loss during the early articulation period. If so, habit strength can cause misarticulations that were originally the result of sensory hearing loss to persist. When this is suspected, sensory and perceptual training should be emphasized. Another diagnostic problem concerns children with intermittent middle-ear disease and therefore, in all probability, fluctuating hearing loss. Their functional hearing efficiency is not accurately represented by a threshold measured when they are well, since at other times they may have a mild to moderate hearing loss.

The patterns of hearing loss differ. A *flat* audiogram is one in which the loss for all frequencies is approximately equal. Impaired sensitivity between 400 and 2,000 Hz, which is sometimes called the *resonance range,* interferes with recognition and discrimination of the *vowels, diphthongs,* and [r], [l], [j], [m], [n], [ŋ], and [w]. High frequency sounds are also affected, and to a relatively greater extent for any given loss, since these sounds carry less acoustic energy and are thus less audible than the low frequency sounds. Losses in the *high frequency range,* which extends from 2,000 to 8,000 Hz approximately, will impair recognition and discrimination of the *fricative, affricate,* and *plosive* sounds. A *high frequency loss* is characterized by a sloping audiogram in which the defect is confined to, or is relatively greater in, frequencies above 2,000 Hz. Losses confined to the frequencies below 400 Hz have relatively little effect on speech understanding, except for some difficulty in distinguishing voiced and voiceless sounds.

44   A further discussion of the effect of *regional hearing loss* on recognition and discrimination of the various speech sounds will be found in Streng, *et al.* (297).

Hearing losses in children are most often *conductive,* a type in which some pathological condition prevents transmission of sound through the outer or middle ears. Middle-ear infection of some kind *(otitis media),* with or without earache *(otalgia)* or draining ears *(otorrhea)* is by far the most common cause. An acute ear infection may be followed by *serous otitis media,* in which the middle ear remains filled with fluid which has not drained, and subsequently becomes thickened. This condition is often overlooked because there are no symptoms perceptible to the layman, yet hearing may be impaired. Hearing loss is not always present in *otitis media,* although losses up to 40 dB are the rule. A flat audiogram is typical. Repeated infection can cause a permanent impairment, so that prompt and vigorous medical treatment is imperative—and fortunately it is usually successful.

Sensorineural hearing loss, although less common, causes most of the severe hearing losses of early infancy and childhood. Sensorineural losses are of two types: *cochlear,* in which case the dysfunction is in the end organ of hearing in the inner ear, or *retrocochlear,* in which case the dysfunction is in the neural system beyond the cochlea, specifically the auditory nerve, the auditory tract, or the brain centers of hearing. Sensorineural losses are caused by a wide variety of pathologies of pre- and postnatal origin, and there is little medical treatment. The audiograms can be flat, but a high frequency loss is more common. There are also a number of conditions covered by the term *dysacusis,* in which the ability to recognize speech is impaired even though sensitivity is normal or nearly so.

45   See also Davis and Silverman (68).

Kinesthesis

This sense conveys information about the direction and extent of muscle movements and is necessary for the learning and control of motor activities. It is important to "get the feel" of swinging a golf club, or any other skilled act. In the absence of kinesthesia it is impossible to execute movements correctly, except insofar as vision, touch, or some other cue can be used for control. Disturbances in kinesthesia occur in a number of neuropathologies, but little is known about differences in kinesthetic sensibility which fall within the normal range. It is possible that functional disabilities in kinesthesia can cause defective articulation.

46   The studies of McCrosky (178) and Ringel (238) are of interest in this connection.

Touch

Tactile cues unquestionably contribute to phonetic learning and articulation control. One can, for instance, feel many of the contacts at the point of articulation, as when the lower lip is held against the cutting edge of the upper teeth for [f] or [v]. The friction of the breath stream can also be felt, as, for example, when [s] or [ʃ] is articulated. Normally the speaker is not conscious of either kinesthetic or tactile sensations during speech production, but he can learn to attend to them through sensory training, if this is needed. Defects in tactile sensibility as causes of disorders of articulation are hard to identify, however, and the whole matter needs further exploration. Tactile *anethesias* or *paresthesias* are common in stroke victims, children with cerebral palsy, and numerous other neuropathologies in which articulation is also disordered. Research has shown that the elimination of tactile sensations by anesthesia causes profound changes in articulation. To what extent functional tactile defects may be involved in "nonorganic" conditions is impossible to say.

47   Bosma (34) has edited an important symposium on oral tactile sensibility which contains information having many implications for disordered articulation.

Perceptual Deficits

Perception is the process by which the organism selects, organizes, and interprets information made available by the senses. Without some such process the world would be too chaotic to cope with. Words, for instance, would be no more than indistinguishable sounds—a conglomerate of hisses, pops, and moans—if we could not organize them into recognizable words, phrases, and sentences. Perceptual defect is a frequent—some would say the most frequent—cause of learning disabilities, including those of the kind in which we are interested.

A first aspect of perception, termed *primitive perceptual organization,* is critical for the acquisition and maintenance of normal articulation. In this process, the organism, presumably through learning (although there are *nativistic* theories), structures incoming stimuli in various ways. A second aspect of perception involves *symbolic* factors through which any given *percept* not only has primitive organization, but also takes on meaning within the context of one's *apperceptive mass,* or past experience. Thus, primitive perceptual organization might permit an individual to match two objects placed before him, but leave him unable to grasp their "meaning" without calling on symbolic processes. This latter aspect of perception is, of course, intimately related to language reception.

The elements of primitive perceptual organization are *grouping, closure, figure-ground effect,* and *constancy.* Through the process of grouping incoming stimuli are perceived as being "together" or "separate." For instance, if a syllable were to be repeated three times at half-second intervals then again after a two-second interval (la-la-la——la), we would hear the first three as being together and the fourth as separate. This kind of structuring is a requisite for the perception of speech. Closure leads us to supply missing information, so that a word incompletely heard can nevertheless be recognized. The figure-ground effect enables one to organize and relate incoming stimuli in such a way that a *figure,* to which we attend specifically, takes form against a total background. We can thus recognize speech against a background of noise and other competing stimuli because we have the perceptual capacity to maintain appropriate figure-ground relationships. Constancy makes it possible to perceive things as the "same" despite actual differences. A spoken word, for instance, varies considerably in its acoustic make-up from one time to another, yet it is perceived as the same word under all conditions.

Perceptual defects, particularly in hearing, are still incompletely understood. Nevertheless, by calling on clinical observation, such research findings as are available, and the general facts about normal perception, it is possible to draw a number of inferences on which to base the diagnosis and treatment of speech disorders. Both clinical and research literature make it clear that perceptual deficit is a primary symptom of neurological impairment in children and adults; indeed, the "brain-damaged" child is sometimes labeled the "perceptually-handicapped" child. Although perceptual disabilities are an accepted symptom of pathology, there have been no definitive investigations on individual differences among normals in perceptual function. Nevertheless, as a clinical hypothesis we may assume that these differences exist and that they probably differ only in degree from the known perceptual defects that occur in neurological impairment.

Deficits in primitive perceptual organization are probably most closely related to disorders of articulation. The inability to maintain appropriate figure-ground relationships, which is an established phenomenon in the neurologically impaired, can certainly impair articulation learning. To be perceived, the acoustic signals of spoken language must first be structured against the background of other sounds in most listening conditions. Next, finer figure-ground relationships must be established if individual features—words, syllables, and sounds—are to be distinguished in the complex configurations of speech. The confusion that confronts anyone with a figure-ground defect was expressed by an adult with brain damage who complained that speech was "just a jumble of sound." As would be expected, this disability becomes more marked as the complexity of the stimuli increases. There are several possible reasons for the *idiolalia* of brain-injured children, but perceptual defect of this type is certainly among them. Difficulties in phonetic anlaysis and synthesis may also be related to this kind of perceptual defect.

> 48   Unfortunately there are no definitive diagnostic tests for figure-ground defects in audition, but for a description of those in the area of vision, and for a general treatment of figure-ground defects, consult Strauss and Lehtinen (295) and Strauss and Kephart (296).

Comments on other aspects of perception must be still more speculative. Grouping is unquestionably essential for accurate speech reception, since its absence would leave the listener unable to recognize the existence of configurations of sound. Short *auditory memory span* may, at least in some children, be a deficit in perception rather than memory. Poor *phonetic discrimination* must also be considered a form of auditory imperception in some cases.

Interestingly, closure and constancy, although necessary for speech perception, may actually interfere with the fine discrimination of sounds that facilitates articulation learning, since these perceptual capacities allow one to recognize words without being aware of their full acoustic characteristics.

> 49   Darley (65) has further information on both auditory memory span and phonetic discrimination.

Some neuropathologists recognize a perceptual disorder called loss of *sensitivity* or *reactivity*. It consists of an inabilty to attend to stimuli, without significant sensory loss. This disorder may explain why children with known neurological impairment do not respond to loud speech or other sounds, or do so intermittently, even though they have no actual hearing loss. This is so common that such children are frequently diagnosed as deaf or hard of hearing. Inconsistency of response is typical; the child may pay no attention to a shout, but turn his head when a door is closed softly behind his back.

50   See Schlesinger (259) for a description of this and other disorders of perception.

Although we have discussed mostly auditory perception because of its importance in speech reception, the input at any given time is a mixture of auditory, tactile, proprioceptive, visual, and other sensations. Sorting these out into meaningful patterns imposes greater demands on perception than if there were only one modality and renders the organism more vulnerable to dysfunction. There is considerable evidence that the neurologically impaired may be subject to *intersensory interference* because they cannot deal adequately with stimuli arriving simultaneously through more than one channel. This is essentially the same thing that causes a normal person to close his eyes in order to listen more carefully to a faint sound. People who have such a perceptual deficit must be trained, at least initially, through a single sensory modality—the one that is least impaired, if this can be discovered.

DELAYED MATURATION

Maturation is the process by which an organism, through growth and development, acquires the potential for progressively more elaborate, complex, and versatile behavior. Learning and maturation are complementary. Activities such as walking and talking are learned, but only when the child has reached a state of readiness. He was not ready at birth, and no amount of teaching could have made him walk or talk until he had the capacity to do so. Given the opportunity, he might actually do some of the things we ordinarily think of as learned behavior through maturation alone. Other behaviors, including talking, depend on both maturation and learning. Maturation of physical and psychological capacities underlies all kinds of behavior. Slowness or complete failure to achieve readiness can be responsible for many developmental anomalies of childhood, including speech disorders. The border between functional and organic is ill-defined in this case, but a diagnosis of maturational delay implies, or at least raises the hope, that further growth and development will enhance the child's potential for learning.

The determinants of speech readiness were discussed earlier. They are all, of course, intimately interrelated in a total growth pattern.

51   An excellent single reference for maturation is Mussen, Conger, and Kagan (206).

The perfection of neuromuscular mechanisms is a prime necessity for articulation. An infant is born with the basic central nervous system centers and pathways which will serve him thoughout life, but they do not become functional until certain postnatal growth processes take place. The neonate is, so to speak, like a complex electronic machine whose parts are all present, but whose wiring is incomplete. It is therefore capable of only limited functions, and will not be fully operational until the circuits are finished. In the clinical diagnosis of children with certain pathologies the neurologist may find *release signs,* such as the persistence of primitive reflexes (the *Babinski,* for instance) which are normally abolished when higher centers, after the completion of conducting pathways, take command.

Suckling, swallowing, and respiratory reflexes are present at birth, but circuits for the articulation derivatives of these inborn movements are not. They develop rapidly, however, and the basic motor skills for speech, although not perfected, are present in the normal child no later than his second birthday. Neuromuscular maturation is reflected in babbling. Further maturation, augmented by learning, produces vocal play, jargon, and eventually the early linguistic stages of speech development. The process is not completed until the child has learned all of the sounds of speech, normally between the seventh and eighth birthdays.

Delayed neuromuscular maturation is not always easy to identify. The most reliable sign is a generalized lag in motor development—the child is behind schedule in sitting, standing, walking, and so on. A diminished activity level, little or no crying in early infancy, and limited babbling are all reasons for suspicion. Usually any neuromuscular retardation is generalized so that all kinds of motor responses are slow to appear or reduced in amount, but occasionally only the sound-making activities seem to be affected. Information about the infant's suckling and swallowing is of great interest, since those who prove slow in developing articulation skills not uncommonly have a history of feeding difficulties and later have such symptoms as inability to chew and swallow firm-textured foods such as meat.

52 A standard reference on diagnosis of developmental retardation is Gesell and Amatruda (101).

It is not always clear what causes lags in neuromuscular development. Brain damage, sometimes no more than minimal in degree, is certainly one cause. Poor physical status and unsatisfactory growth in early childhood is another. Slower maturation in boys than in girls is to be expected, and there appear to be inborn differences among children for which no ready explanation can be offered. Some of these are unquestionably due to undiagnosed central nervous system damage, but others must be presumed to have a genetic basis. Finally, psychosocial forces are by no means unimportant, for even in the first few weeks of an infant's life emotional deprivation may depress his activity level and hence his motor development. In extreme cases the result may be *marasmus,* or an actual physical wasting.

So far as training is concerned, increased motor activities—including chewing, sucking, swallowing, and babbling exercises—are indicated if slow neuromuscular maturation is suspected. Large muscle skills assist the acquisition of fine coordinations. A key judgment must be made about the level of motor readiness with the understanding that even in cases of severe motor disability, such as cerebral palsy, growth may improve the child's neuromuscular potential.

Compared to his motor abilities, the sensory endowment an infant brings into the world is relatively good. His senses are not as acute as they will be in a few months, but hearing, kinesthesia, touch, and vision mature rapidly. Hearing has been demonstrated in unborn infants, and the newborn are responsive to sound, although acuity is not good in the first few days.

Variations in the intensity and duration of sounds readily evoke changes in behavior in the neonatal period. Pitch discrimination appears to develop after a few months, but must be present before the emergence of inflected vocal play, which, in a normally developing infant, is in the latter half of his first year. Localizing responses to sound can be reliably elicited in infants with normal hearing at six months or before. The best available evidence suggests that by 24 months a child has essentially a full complement of sensory capacities in audition.

53   Further information on early auditory behavior can be found in
Hardy (114).

Kinesthesis and touch are also present in more than a rudimentary form at birth and mature quite soon thereafter. It appears, then, that at least minimal sensory readiness for speech is normally present at 12 months, or shortly before. Aside from actual sensory defect, the existence of lags in sensory maturation—and their causes, if they do exist—remains somewhat conjectural. Central nervous system impairment, poor physical status and growth, inborn individual differences, and deprivation are probably etiologic factors, but the whole matter is obscure so far as clinical diasgnosis is concerned.

The maturation of perception and of the circuitry mediating control of articulation movements, language formulation, and other facets of linguistic behavior takes place over an extended period of time. The age at which phonetic skills are perfected—seven to eight years—can be considered the time when both the primary effector and higher integrative neural networks have matured, and any increase in motor speech potential after this age will be minimal in normal children. Unless significant maturational delay is presumed, if growth is continuing, misarticulations which persist must be attributed to habit strength, psychosocial factors, or some other etiology. In a larger sense, maturation of perception and of the capacity for linguistic behavior are part of the higher psychological development that continues into at least the second decade of life.

Brain damage is the best understood cause of the disorders of communication that involve perception, operation of the higher integrative motor circuits, or the language processes (*agnosia,* *apraxia,* and *aphasia,* respectively). When comparable symptoms occur as an apparent result of the failure of normal function to develop—which is essentially what is meant by *developmental aphasia*—the etiology is less definite. Once more we suppose that some cases spring from undiagnosed exogenous brain damage, and that others are genetically based defects of growth and development. The disorders are sometimes said to be *idiopathic,* or of unknown etiology, although they still are assumed to have a neural basis since the symptoms are accepted as behavioral signs of neurological impairment. One can, however, ignore the question of etiology and say that these disorders represent a failure of the brain to develop *functional integration.* Although somewhat beyond the scope of our immediate concern with articulation, the disorders of language that are associated with neurological signs such as lack of cerebral dominance, mirror writing, reversals in reading, and other signs of functional disorganization in the central nervous system are of great interest.

54   Both the early work of Orton (217) and some of the recent discussions of neural organization in the book by Schlesinger (259) bear on these points.

IN MORPHOGENIC DISORDERS OF ARTICULATION PRODUCTION OF THE speech sounds is made difficult or impossible because of some structural abnormality in or about the mouth. Morphogenic disorders of articulation are forms of *dysglossia,* and the structural deformities are usually called *orofacial* defects, or *maxillofacial* defects if only the upper jaw is involved (as in congenital cleft of the lip and jaw). This etiology can be roughly estimated as responsible for 10 to 15 per cent of all articulation cases.

There is no doubt that deviations in the size, shape, and relationship of structures in the peripheral speech mechanism can interfere with production of the speech sounds, but the relationship between mouth structure and articulation is not simple. One person with an orofacial defect will speak normally, while another with what looks

5 *morphologic factors*

like an identical condition will have seriously impaired articulation as a result. Every experienced clinician has seen cases where good speech has been achieved under what would seem to be impossible conditions: when all or part of the tongue has been removed surgically, an open cleft of the palate exists, or the speaker has a gross deformity of the dental arch. On the other hand, slight structural deviations can cause a great deal of trouble for some speakers.

The reasons for these individual differences are not always clear. Of course, there are many ways to produce acoustically acceptable speech sounds, a fact demonstrated by the success of a skilled ventriloquist. The flexibility and agility of the tongue and other articulation muscles make it possible to compensate for deviations in mouth structure, within the limits of individual capabilities. Intelligence and motivation also determine success in compensation. Good hearing is a necessity. With children, the amount of informal teaching they have received is a variable. Anxiety and emotional stress related to either articulation or the defect itself will have an effect. In addition, there is an X factor, a kind of "phonetic aptitude" not yet understood, that affects success in overcoming orofacial defects.

---

55 See either West (331) or Bloomer (33) for a further discussion of these matters.

In deciding whether or not a mouth deformity is a significant factor, each individual must be considered on his own merits. A good rule of thumb is to consider any structural deviation a possible cause of misarticulation, provided the nature of the speech defect is consistent with the deviation. Even if a speaker can, by extraordinary effort, compensate for the defective structure, his difficulty of doing so may impose a real burden on him. Surgical or dental treatment before speech training is the most conservative approach.

Structural deviations can affect articulation in the following ways: (1) interference with contacts between the articulators can cause misarticulation of the labial plosives, labiodentals, lingua-dentals, lingua-alveolars, and linguapalatals; (2) deviations in the mouth surfaces against which the breath stream is normally directed can distort the fricatives; and (3) insufficient palatopharyngeal closure can impair resonance. A diagnostic judgment is made only after a phonetic inventory in which the acoustic characteristics of the defective sounds are carefully considered. One then decides whether or not, in view of the manner in which the sound in question is produced, there *could* be a relationship between the faulty structure and the acoustic characteristics of the defective sound. For example, even the most aggravated dental malocclusion could not account for a [w]/[r] substitution, but it could distort any of the sibilant sounds, particularly if the anterior segments of the upper dental arch are involved.

The common orofacial defects that can contribute to articulation disorders are grouped in four categories: (1) congenital cleft of the lip and palate, (2) other congenital deformities, (3) dental malocclusions, and (4) acquired orofacial defects.

Congenital cleft of the lip and palate

The most frequent of the serious orofacial defects is congenital cleft of the lip and palate. Estimates of the incidence of this condition range from one in 600-800 live births to one in 2,000 births. Speech problems are almost always present. The speech pathologist has two functions in the habilitation of these children: first, to cooperate with other specialists in planning surgical, dental, or other measures, and, second, to provide speech training if necessary.

Congenital cleft of the lip and palate result from a failure in growth of the embryo and fetus. In cleft lip and palate the infant is born with splits at certain points in the lip and in the roof of the mouth where the parts would normally have fused. Traditionally, these abnormalities have been considered hereditary, but in recent years considerable evidence has been accumulated suggesting that these embryonic growth failures result from exogenous influences which interfere with normal prenatal development. These studies imply that the time may come when these and other birth defects can be prevented by proper prenatal care.

> 56   A full treatment of all aspects of cleft lip and palate will be found in Westlake and Rutherford (334) and Morley (199).

The various forms of clefts of the lip and palate are summarized in the following outline:

1. Clefts of the *lip*.
   a. *Unilateral* or *bilateral*—on one side only (either right or left), or on both sides.
   b. *Partial* or *complete*—partial clefts of the lip extend upward from the vermilion border of the lip, but not as far as the floor of the nose; complete clefts do extend into the floor of the nose, entirely separating the anterior central portion of the upper lip (*prolabium*) from the adjacent tissue of the face.
2. Clefts of the *lip* and *jaw* involve both the lip and jaw (but not the hard palate).
   a. *Unilateral* or *bilateral*—on one side only (right or left), or on both sides.
   b. *Partial* or *complete*—partial clefts of the lip segment are as described above; accompanying jaw clefts involve the lower margin of the gum ridge (*alveolar process*) and extend upward, but do not go into the floor of the nose; complete clefts do go into the floor of the nose, thus completely separating the anterior central portion of the upper jaw (*premaxilla*) from the adjacent portion of the jaw. (Clefts of the lip or jaw may occur separately.)
3. Clefts of the *soft palate* (*velar* clefts).
   a. *Partial* or *complete*—partial clefts extend forward some distance into the soft palate from its posterior border (thus splitting the *uvula*), but do not reach the bony palate; complete clefts do extend to the posterior border of the bony palate.
4. Clefts of the *hard palate*.
   a. *Partial* or *complete*—here there is always a complete cleft of the soft palate; a partial cleft of the bony palate extends some distance forward from its posterior border, but does not reach the premaxilla; complete clefts of the hard palate do extend forward to its anterior boundary at the *incisive fossa* just behind the premaxilla. The two halves of the bony palate, which is made up of the *palatine processes* of the right and left *maxillary bones,* are thus completely separated.
5. *Lip-jaw-palate* clefts—a combination of the forms described above,

usually with complete cleft of the soft and hard palates; the lip-jaw segment may show a unilateral or bilateral, and partial or complete cleft.

Any of the foregoing clefts may vary in width, according to the amount of deficiency in tissue growth. A relatively rare form of *median* lip-jaw cleft consists of a split at the midline through the vertical depression in the upper lip (*philtrum*) and the jaw directly behind this point. Of great interest to the speech consultant are *submucous clefts* in which muscular or bony tissue is cleft, but the overlying mucous membrane is not. Because there is no easily seen opening, this condition is often overlooked and, if the soft palate is involved, typical cleft-palate speech may result. Dental malocclusions and cosmetic defects are common in all of the conditions described above, but are particularly prominent in lip-jaw and lip-jaw-palate clefts. A congenitally short soft palate without cleft or associated with submucous cleft or open cleft is a frequent finding.

In assessing the cleft-palate individual and planning his treatment, it is helpful to distinguish between the *primary* and *secondary* speech defects. Those considered primary arise directly from *velar incompetence* (also called *velopharyngeal* or *palatopharyngeal incompetence*) and from dental deformities associated with clefts of the palate or jaw. Velar incompetence, which allows air to flow into the *nasopharynx* and *nasal passages* during speech, leads to *hypernasal* vocal quality and insufficient *intraoral breath pressure* for the plosives, fricatives, and affricates. A nasal fricative sound is often an undesirably conspicuous feature of cleft-palate speech. Any jaw deformity will affect articulation according to the general principles discussed at the beginning of this chapter. Appropriate surgical or dental treatment, or both, is usually required before speech training for primary defects.

Secondary defects are related only indirectly to velar incompetence or dental deformities. The distinction is a simple one but must be made with care, since secondary speech defects do not call for surgical or dental treatment before training. Needless surgery or dental treatment to improve speech is occasionally prescribed when the true cause of the defective articulation is not fully appreciated. The major causes of secondary defects include: (1) hearing loss, which is present in many cases; (2) aspects of the orofacial defect that indirectly cause functional misarticulations that would not be improved by surgery, prosthesis, or dental treatment; (3) functional weakness of the musculature responsible for palatopharyngeal closure; and (4) delay or defect in the development of articulation skills caused by the psychosocial factors that are likely to be associated with a speech handicap. There is always the possibility that a person with a cleft palate might have an articulation disorder unrelated to the cleft.

For a full description of the comprehensive and prolonged treatment and training these children require see the texts cited earlier. Generally speaking, complete habilitation calls for extensive and coordinated treatment including general medical care, plastic surgery, otological treatment, prosthodontia, orthodontia, and speech training. Beyond these, the cleft-palate individual may need special education, psychotherapy, vocational counselling, and similar measures. Habilitation is difficult and costly, but it is remarkably successful if the program is good. The speech pathologist plays an important role.

OTHER CONGENITAL ANOMALIES

Congenital orofacial defects other than cleft palate and lip are much less frequent. Possibly the best known anomaly of the tongue is *ankyglossia* or "tongue-tie," a condition in which mobility of the front of the tongue is limited. There are two forms of this defect. In the first, the *lingual frenum*—a "cord" running from the floor of the mouth to the under side of the tongue—inserts closer to the tongue tip than it should, thus preventing extension and elevation of the front part of the tongue. Incidentally, a mistaken diagnosis of tongue-tie may be made in very young infants; the frenum appears to have an insertion too far forward, but this condition is corrected as the tongue tip develops. The practice of routinely clipping the lingual frenum was once carried out in some hospitals, but is now rare. Nevertheless, a case history noting that the child was tongue-tied until his frenum was cut should be interpreted with caution.

In the other form of ankyglossia the muscular "root" of the tongue actually inserts at or near the tip, so that mobility is distinctly impaired. Surgery is necessary if there are any functional problems. In either type of ankyglossia all sounds for which the tongue must be thrust forward or the tip elevated are threatened, although many children compensate well. As usual, a decision on the effect of tongue-tie on articulation depends on the nature of the child's phonetic errors and, of course, how severely movements of the tongue are restricted. Ordinarily one assumes that there is sufficient mobility for speech production if the tongue tip can be brought far enough forward to rest between the upper and lower teeth.

Sometimes the tongue is disproportionately large in comparison with the size of the mandible, a condition called *macroglossia.* Such a situation may be congenital, but it may also be associated with a pathology causing *edema* (swelling). As might be anticipated, *oral inaccuracy* is a typical articulation defect, not only because of tongue size, but also because the movements tend to be flaccid. Lingual fissures may appear unusually deep in macroglossia. A *bifid* or split tongue occurs, but is rare. A tongue of normal size in an unusually small mandible should not be mistaken for macroglossia. For speech purposes, the size relationship between the tongue and upper dental arch is most critical.

There are several other orofacial defects of congenital origin, which, like cleft lip and palate, fall into the category of *branchial arch* anomalies (sometimes called *branchial arch dysplasias*). Surgical and dental treatment similar to that for cleft lip and palate is generally needed. The nature and severity of any associated defects of articulation will, of course, depend on the individual and the characteristics of his deformity. As with cleft lip and palate, the origin of these other birth defects is not entirely clear, but they also are presumed to be either developmental growth failures or genetically based. A speech pathologist should be involved in the total treatment of most of these cases.

One such orofacial defect, called the *Pierre Robin* syndrome, may have serious speech consequences. This syndrome consists of aggravated *micrognathia* or underdevelopment of the mandible, often (but not necessarily) accompanied by cleft palate. There is an immediate hazard at birth of strangulation because the tongue tends to drop back into the infant's throat. To prevent this the tongue tip was once sutured to the inner surface of the lower lip, although better techniques have been devised more recently. This restriction of movement, along with the small narrow lower jaw and possible cleft palate can have a catastrophic effect on the child's articulation learning. Growth of the lower jaw is usually quite good so that the tongue can be freed in due course, but there may be significant interference with early speech development.

The *Treacher-Collins syndrome,* sometimes called *congenital multifacial dystrophy,* is somewhat less of a direct threat to articulation, although not always, but it does cause severe cosmetic defects. In this condition there are deficiencies in the *malar prominence* (cheekbone) and *infraorbital ridge* (lower border of the eye pits), so that the area looks flattened or pushed in; *micrognathia;* a notching of the lower eyelids with slanting of the *palpebral folds* (above the eyes); and *ear deformities* that may cause severe hearing impairment. There may also be other congenital deformities, including cleft palate.

Facial clefts (other than cleft lip) occur in varying forms and sometimes cause articulation difficulties. A *maxillomandibular cleft* extends horizontally back from the corner of the mouth toward the ear, usually on both sides but sometimes on one side only. Here there has been a failure of fusion between the mandibular and maxillary processes, which are the *anlagen* (embryonic forerunners) for the cheeks and other structures. Lip movement is sometimes poor for speech even when plastic surgery has been successful in improving the child's appearance. In *oblique facial cleft* a split extends through the upper lip lateral to the nostril, sometimes as far as the eye. Both appearance and speech are severely affected. A *mandibular cleft* (with or without bifid tongue) separates the two halves of the lower jaw.

Defects of vocal resonance are sometimes a fringe problem in some of the congenital deformities of the nose. These include: midline *nose cleft* which is very infrequent in its complete form, although separation of the *septal cartilages* at the tip of the nose is not; a complete absence of nasal structures; *hump nose,* an apparent enlargement of the upper portion; and *saddle nose,* in which there is a marked depression above the tip. There is a wide variety of congenital conditions that partially or completely obstruct the nasal passages and may cause later problems for voice and hearing.

There are a few mouth deformities not previously mentioned that can interfere with speech function. The normal limits for lip size are rather wide, but excessively large lips, called *macrocheilia,* can have some effect on function, mostly because the labial muscles tend to be flaccid. When this structure folds upon itself horizontally, it looks like a double upper lip. Children born with *astomia,* or absence of an oral opening, usually do not survive, but both *macrostomia,* an unusually large mouth opening, and *microstomia,* the opposite, may be encountered. The size of the interior of the mouth may be enlarged or reduced and articulation consequently impaired. *Hyperplastic gingival tissue* (excessively developed gums) may also interfere. In one such case space in the lower dental arch was so limited that the child's tongue could not lie flat on the floor of his mouth. In another, space in the upper arch was similarly restricted. Unfortunately this tissue tends to proliferate once more after trimming.

No general rules can be made about the speech complications of these congenital deformities. Each case must be studied individually and imaginative training techniques devised when mouth architecture prevents the development of good speech. Fortunately these birth defects do not occur often, but when they do they present a great challenge to the surgical and dental specialists. The speech pathologist should be able to capitalize on their treatment if a speech defect is part of the child's problem.

57   For a full treatment of birth defects, consult Mayer and Swanker (173).

DENTAL MALOCCLUSIONS

Dental malocclusions threaten speech when they make it difficult or impossible to achieve the necessary acoustic conditions. From the standpoint of orthodontia, a dental malocclusion is some deviation in the occlusal relationship of the maxillary and mandibular teeth. Criteria for diagnosing the presence and severity of a malocclusion include cosmetic considerations, and the function of the teeth in mastication and articulation.

Most orthodontists use the *Angle* classification of malocclusions, and an understanding of it is useful for the speech pathologist. In this scheme the upper first molars (six-year molars) are used as fixed points of reference, and the types of malocclusions are based on the relationship of the lower first molars to the corresponding upper teeth. Following are the major types of malocclusions:

Class I—Neutrocclusion

In this class the molars are in a normal relationship, with the *mesial buccal cusp* of the maxillary tooth fitting into the buccal groove of the lower first molar when the jaws are in a closed position.[1] In neutrocclusion the molars occlude normally, but there

[1] Molars have four projections or *cusps,* one at each "corner" of the occlusal surface of the tooth; the *groove* is, of course, the indentation into which the cusp of an opposing molar fits when they are in normal contact. In dental terminology the surfaces of teeth are identified as follows: *buccal,* toward the cheek; *lingual,* toward the tongue; and *labial,* toward the lip (when referring to the cuspids and incisors). The terms *mesial* and *distal* mean toward and away from the midline, respectively, but since the midline of the dental arch lies between the two central incisor teeth, *distal* and *mesial* may be thought of as approximately the same as "posterior" and "anterior" when the relationship of the molars is under discussion.

is some abnormality in the relationships of teeth in the anterior portion of the arch.

Class II—Distocclusion

In this class the lower first molar is *distal* to (behind) its normal position in relation to the upper first molar. A number of subclasses are provided in the detailed Angle classification, but in general the lower jaw is receding, giving the individual a *retrognathic* profile. The upper front teeth bite further ahead of the lowers than is normal (*overbite* in nontechnical language). Often the upper arch is narrow, with a high palatal vault.

Class III—Mesiocclusion

In this type of occlusion the lower first molar is forward from, or *mesial* to, its proper position in relation to the corresponding upper molar. This creates *underbite* with a protruding lower jaw and a *prognathic profile*. The disparity in size between the upper and lower jaws may be hereditary (and is sometimes related to racial characteristics), but it is also often a feature of cleft lip and palate because of a bony deficiency in the upper arch. Tongue size and position are ordinarily appropriate to the size of the mandibular arch, which is a point of interest in connection with the articulation problems of these cases.

In addition to disturbances in the relationship of the upper to the lower dental arches, individual teeth may be *malposed* in various ways. They may be tipped inward (*lingual*) or outward (*buccal* or *labial*), or rotated on a vertical axis, as commonly happens with a lateral incisor in clefts of the jaw. They may erupt in other anomalous positions, which is also common in clefts of the jaw. Teeth may be missing, either because they have been lost or because the tooth buds from which they should have developed are absent. Malposed or missing teeth may create unusual irregularities and openings in the dental surfaces against which the breath stream is directed for certain speech sounds and thus impair their acoustic qualities.

In what is called an *anterior openbite* the incisors do not meet and overlap as they should when the molars are in occlusion or when the mandible is in resting position. There is instead an abnormal opening in the anterior part of the bite which can affect the quality of the sibilants. A *closed bite* is the opposite condition, in which the upper incisors project too far downward over the lowers, sometimes so far that the lower teeth are hidden. Closed bite does not usually cause misarticulations except in extreme cases. *Crossbite* is a general term for a condition in which the teeth bite inside or outside of their normal position, and is also not a serious threat to articulation unless sufficiently severe.

> 58   Refer to Bloomer (33) for an extensive treatment of the relation between dental malocclusions and articulation.

Most orthodontists regard heredity, growth and nutritional deficiencies, and bad mouth habits as the causes of malocclusions. Bad mouth habits are those that create unnatural pressures on teeth and thus move them from their normal positions. Thumbsucking, lip-biting, reading with one's chin resting in his hands, and similar practices are examples. Recently there has been great interest in a condition variously called *tongue thrust, reverse swallow, infantile swallow,* and *orofacial muscle imbalance.* Briefly, this is a disturbance in swallowing patterns in which the tongue is thrust forward against or between the anterior central teeth. Swallowing is also accompanied by certain abnormal contractions of the facial musculature which the individual finds necessary to facilitate swallowing. The resulting abnormal pressures, which occur several times each minute as one swallows reflexively to clear the mouth of accumulated saliva, will, many orthodontists think, contribute to anterior openbite, labioversion of the anterior central teeth, and other conditions. The cause of tongue thrust remains obscure, but the general opinion is that this habit is caused by the lack of physiologically normal feeding movements in most bottle-fed babies. Some suspect the pattern is inborn.

Abnormal articulation movements appear to be part of this syndrome. There is a generalized forward thrust on the lingual sounds, particularly the sibilants. Protrusive, lateral, and diffuse lisps are often prominent. There is also some laxity and poor control in the musculature of deglutition and articulation, although some of the facial muscles are overdeveloped because of their unusual participation in swallowing. The tongue thrust in speaking, along with that in swallowing, contributes to the abnormal pressures on the teeth. Those who have worked with these children as an adjunct to orthodontic treatment feel that articulation should be trained as well as swallowing. They also report that the swallowing training greatly facilitates articulation training, even to the point that defective sounds may clear up spontaneously, so that the two kinds of therapy are mutually reinforcing. Although still

a subject of some debate, there is now sufficient clinical and research evidence to support the position that tongue thrust is important to the speech pathologist, both theoretically and clinically.

59   Palmer (219) has a general article on this subject, and a good bibliog-
      raphy of other recent titles.

ACQUIRED OROFACIAL DEFECTS

Orofacial defects caused by injury or disease are common, particularly in the adult population, and speech training may be an
essential part of the total treatment. These defects are so miscel-
laneous that there is really no way they can be satisfactorily classified. Again, the mouth structure and muscle function must be
studied carefully in relation to the sounds that are defective. Great
ingenuity may be needed to find nonstandard ways of producing
speech sounds for some of the badly damaged patients.

There are many causes of injury, and the patient may be left
with either minor or major changes in mouth structure after surgical and dental treatment. He may have to learn neuromuscular
adjustments for articulation radically different from those he is
accustomed to, or he may simply need help in adjusting to less
drastic changes in the structure of his mouth and face. Accidental
perforation or tearing of the soft palate sometimes occurs when
children fall with sticks or other objects in their mouths and occasionally under other circumstances. Such cases present the same
problems for the plastic surgeon and speech pathologist as congenital clefts of the palate. The term *pseudo-cleft-palate speech* is
sometimes applied to acquired defects in which voice and articulation resemble that heard in congenital cleft palate.

Perforation of the palate in suppurative disease is not as common as it once was, but cases of this kind are still seen by the
plastic surgeon and often must be referred to the speech pathologist after medical treatment has reached the proper point. Such
cases may also be treated by a dentist who specializes in *maxillofacial prosthetics.* The most common type of disease that can cause
speech problems is a *neoplasm,* particularly cancer. In these cases,
the surgeon often has to remove tissue from the site of the tumor.
Radical dissections that leave the patient severely handicapped
cosmetically and functionally are necessary in severe cases. The
tongue, palate, lip, jaw, or portions of the face may have to be
completely or partially removed, with functional consequences that

can readily be imagined. In less severe cases the cosmetic and functional problems are similar but less acute. When speech training is needed, a program of rehabilitation must be worked out to take maximum advantage of what functional potential remains.

ᘯᘯᘯ

Dysarthria MEANS ANY DISORDER OF ARTICULATION IN WHICH MOVE-
ment is impaired because of some neuropathology which prevents
normal function of the motor circuits of the central nervous system. The observable and audible characteristics vary, but they
have in common some weakness or loss of movement, faulty incoordination, or incorrect execution of movement. The degree to
which speech loses intelligibility and becomes conspicuous is com-
mensurate with the type and severity of the underlying motor
disorder.

For descriptive purposes the neurogenic disorders of articulation
can be divided into (1) *lower motor neuron dysarthria,* in which
there is damage either in the *medulla* or in the *peripheral* motor
nerve fibers; (2) what for want of a better term will be called *upper*

6 *neurophysiological factors*

motor neuron, or *suprasegmental, dysarthria,* in which speech movements are disrupted by those incoordinations characteristic of one
or more of the type of *cerebral palsy* (principally *spasticity, athetosis,* and *ataxia*), and (3) *central dysarthria,* a condition in which
articulation movement is potentially normal, but in which there
is a failure of the higher integrative mechanisms of the brain to
pattern and order these movements into the correct speech responses. This last category is essentially the same as *articulation
apraxia.*

LOWER MOTOR NEURON DYSARTHRIA

The articulation musculature is supplied by cranial nerves whose
nuclei lie in the *bulbar* portion of the brainstem. The nerves are
paired right and left and the motor fibers are *homolateral,* descend-
ing to muscles on the same side. Taken together the two nerves of
a pair make up the lower motor neuron segment or "final common
pathway" through which impulses are channeled for the arousal
of articulation movements. *Upper motor neuron* or *suprasegmental*
systems control the lower motor neuron system and ensure coordinated motion. The cranial nerves for articulation can be summarized briefly as follows:

V. *Trigeminal nerve*—the motor fibers of this nerve stimulate the
muscles of jaw movement. The *tensor palati* is also innervated by
a branch of this nerve.

VII. *Facial nerve*—the motor fibers of this nerve stimulate the musculature of the lips, face, forehead, and scalp.

IX. *Glossopharyngeal nerve,* X. *Vagus nerve,* XI. *Spinal Accessory nerve*—through complex interrelated circuits the motor fibers of these three cranial nerves stimulate the muscles of swallowing, sucking, phonation, and respiration. These muscles are also essential for articulation, of course. In addition, this complex also stimulates the extrinsic muscles of the tongue. This lower motor neuron network is complex, but in general the glossopharyngeal nerve stimulates the pharynx; the vagus nerve stimulates the intrinsic and extrinsic laryngeal muscles, the respiratory muscles, and the palate, and contributes to the stimulation of the pharyngeal muscles; the spinal accessory nerve sends motor fibers to some of the pharyngeal muscles.

XII. *Hypoglossal nerve*—this nerve sends motor fibers to the intrinsic tongue muscles.

Damage to this lower motor neuron system deprives the articulation musculature of its normal innervation, so that the clinical symptoms are either a total absence of movement, or weakness of motion. Muscle tone is reduced or abolished, producing *flaccidity.* Contraction is lost completely if, through disease or injury, either the nucleus of a nerve or its peripheral fibers are rendered totally nonfunctional. Weakness occurs when the nucleus or nerve trunk is partially destroyed.

The exact way in which articulation is impaired depends on the location and extent of the lesion. Weakness or loss of motion can be either unilateral or bilateral, depending on whether the nerve supply is interrupted on one or both sides. Lower motor neuron dysarthria can be *bulbar,* if the lesion is in the brainstem, or *peripheral,* if the lesion is somewhere along the course of the nerve. Each of the peripheral nerve trunks has various branches, so that few or many muscles may be affected, depending on the site of the lesion. Although there are exceptions, bulbar lesions are usually bilateral, and peripheral lesions unilateral. Nuclear (i.e. bulbar) lesions usually result from disease, and peripheral lesions from trauma of some kind.

Bulbar Palsy

In bulbar palsy the nuclei in the brainstem are affected, causing some pattern of disability in the muscles of deglutition, respiration, and laryngeal function. Bulbar palsy is caused by a number of degenerative diseases of the central nervous system, most of them not commonly found in children. When poliomyelitis was relatively frequent, the bulbar form of the disease produced these symptoms during the acute stage, and often left more or less permanent damage. A form of *congenital bulbar palsy* is found in children. Unless the cause is an acute infection, the prognosis for a recovery of motion in the affected muscles is generally not good, but whatever rehabilitation is possible should be undertaken.

60   Ford (90) is offered as a reference on all matters related to pathologies of the nervous system.

In bulbar palsy, the patient has difficulty chewing, swallowing, and sometimes breathing. If laryngeal valving is impaired, a *tracheotomy* is often necessary. Speech in bulbar palsy is reduced in intelligibility because of the loss of motility, sluggishness, and weakness of articulation movements. Vowel formation may be imprecise, but the most marked effect of flaccidity is on the nonsyllabic sounds, particularly those that require lip and front-tongue adjustments. Sounds most seriously affected are typically [hw], [w], [t], [d], [l], [p], and [b], but the other sounds are not spared. If the disorder is slight, the result is *lalling* and *oral inaccuracy;* in severe cases articulation movements may be impossible *(anarthria)*. Speech is often weak in intensity because the respiratory muscles are affected, and vocal inflections and variations in force are reduced. Rate is slower than normal. The voice quality is often hypernasal because of insufficient movement of the palatopharyngeal sphincters.

Speech and other symptoms of *pseudobulbar palsy* are much the same as in bulbar palsy, but the lesion is higher in the brain. It is part of the stroke syndrome in many cases, but is also found in many other kinds of central nervous system disease.

Although not a form of bulbar palsy, *myasthenia gravis* presents some of the same symptoms. Speech movements are weak, sluggish, and imprecise, and the voice is likely to be hypernasal. The facial muscles are also weak in many cases. A distinctive feature of this disease is that the muscles function relatively well when rested, but they fatigue rapidly with repeated contraction. Articulation training is rarely needed in myasthenia gravis since medical treatment is successful in most cases.

Dysarthria Associated with Peripheral Nerve Damage

It is difficult, if not impossible, to catalogue the dysarthric symptoms of peripheral nerve damage because of their variability. Motion is often reduced only on one side, so that compensatory movements of the muscles on the unaffected side may make it possible for the patient to talk quite well. Fortunately, peripheral nerve damage, all things considered, does not affect speech very often.

Facial paralysis from VIIth nerve involvement sometimes impairs articulation slightly because of its effect on the labial sounds. In *Bell's palsy,* one of the more common conditions, usually one side of the face is affected. Although there may be some awkwardness in articulation, these cases are rarely presented for speech training since the disease, an inflammatory process, generally yields to medical treatment or remits spontaneously. Injury can cause facial paralysis, again usually on one side. Damage to the facial nerve happens occasionally in ear surgery. In some cases when the nerve is cut or crushed, regeneration and restoration of function occur in time. Flaccidity and weakness of movement will be the central characteristic in all cases. Drooping of the affected muscles, including *ptosis* of the eyelid, cause an asymmetrical facial appearance if unilateral or a mask-like face if bilateral.

Paralysis or weakness of the tongue musculature produces an effect on speech in accord with the nature and degree of muscle dysfunction. Unilateral involvement of the extrinsic muscles causes the tongue to deviate toward the affected side when it is extended. The tonguetip cannot be raised in XIIth nerve damage, nor can other movements, such as grooving, be accomplished. Any muscle that loses its innervation will atrophy in time, a condition that is particularly noticeable in *hemiatrophy* of the tongue (atrophy on one side). Weakness due to denervation of the palatal muscles is not unusual, and movement is often asymmetrical in these cases. This condition sometimes follows tonsillectomy or palate surgery, although in the latter case a congenital abnormality of innervation is also to be suspected. Tonsillectomy sometimes reveals a previously unrecognized paralysis of the palate. Palatal weakness causes hypernasality, nasal air loss, and underarticulation.

A special note should be made about laryngeal nerve paralysis. Because of its course downward along the side of the neck where it makes a "U-turn" and heads upward near the treachea, the *recurrent laryngeal nerve* is unusually vulnerable in neck injury. It may also be damaged during surgery on the neck, particularly operations on the thyroid. All of the intrinsic muscles of the larynx except the cricothroid are supplied by this nerve. There is some variability in effects of recurrent laryngeal nerve lesions, but there is usually a unilateral or bilateral *adductor paralysis* of the vocal folds. If the paralysis is unilateral, the only vocal symptom is a slight breathiness; if bilateral, the patient becomes *aphonic*—he has no voice. Under some circumstances this partial or complete loss of voice is replaced after an interval of weeks or months by an *abductor paralysis* of the vocal folds in which one or both become fixed at the midline. *Stridor* (noisy inhalation) and *dyspnea* (difficulty in breathing) ensue. If the reduced oxygen supply threatens the patient's health, surgery is performed which usually leaves him with a permanent dysphonia. Vigorous vocal exercises may sometimes restore at least partial function in cases of adductor paralysis.

The prognosis for articulation training in cases of lower motor neuron dysarthria must always be guarded. Spontaneous improvement occurs in some cases, but usually both nuclear and peripheral damage leave an irreversible loss of function. Compensatory movements, if not developed spontaneously, can be taught in some cases of unilateral involvement. In other physical disabilities substitute motion is sometimes possible, for example, shoulder movements can compensate for an inability to contract the extensor muscles of the arm. Unfortunately this principle does not have much application to articulation movements. What can be done, and it sometimes results in significant speech improvement, is to give the patient self-monitoring skills and provide a high level of motivation for him to achieve the best level of function permitted by his basic lack of motility. Drill on the speech sounds may improve articulation even though it does not effect any basic change in motility.

Upper motor neuron or suprasegmental dysarthria

In *upper motor neuron* or *suprasegmental dysarthria* the higher motor control circuitry of the brain is not functioning normally because of injury or disease, with the result that both articulation and other voluntary and automatic movements are incoordinate or defective in various ways. Flaccidity of the kind found in lower motor neuron disorders may be present, but the most prominent symptom is *incorrect* movement rather than weakness or absence of motion. Upper motor neuron dysarthrias associated with cerebral palsy are frequently encountered by the speech pathologist. Although classifications differ, five forms of cerebral palsy are usually described: *spasticity, athetosis* (or *dyskinesia*), *ataxia, tremor,* and *rigidity.* Of these the first three account for most of the cases in which there is an articulation disorder. Mixed types of cerebral palsy are also found.

61   In a volume in this series McDonald and Chance (181) present a comprehensive treatment of all phases of cerebral palsy with which the speech pathologist must be concerned. References on special topics will be found in their bibliography.

Spastic Dysarthria

In spastic dysarthria articulation movements are slow, labored or effortful, and inaccurate. The affected muscles are *hypertonic,* that is, they have increased muscle tone or are "overcontracted." The hypertonicity is generally thought to result from the loss of the inhibitory control normally exercised by higher centers on the *stretch reflex,* and an associated breakdown in *reciprocal innervation.* A stretch reflex, as the names implies, is a reflexive contraction that occurs when a muscle is stretched. A familiar example is the knee jerk in which striking the patellar tendon just below the knee cap results in contraction of the quadriceps muscle to which the tendon is attached, causing the leg to kick forward. This and other *tendon reflexes* are usually tested in a routine medical examination to check the integrity of the underlying neural mechanisms.

In a normal organism the stretch reflex helps to maintain posture, but it must be inhibited in order to carry out actions that require an alteration in the dynamically balanced contractions of the postural musculature. *Reciprocal innervation* is a neural mechanism which inhibits the contraction of the *antogonist* muscle when an *agonist* is contracted. In flexion of the arm, for instance, contraction of the agonist (in this case the biceps) inhibits the contraction of the antogonist (the triceps), so that there is no extensor interference with the flexor action. In a spastic arm, however, the threshold for the stretch reflex is pathologically lowered, and contraction of the flexor causes the slightly stretched extensor to contract also. The result is a generalized contraction of these arm muscles; movement is slower than normal and inaccurate because the muscles are working against each other.

There are many unanswered questions about the pathological basis for spastic symptoms, but it is generally believed that they are caused by damage to the pyramidal system. Spasticity is essentially a *release* symptom, that is, a symptom that occurs when more primitive mechanisms are not held under the control of functionally higher motor circuits. Other release signs diagnostic of spasticity are abnormal persistence of certain primitive righting reflexes, the Babinski sign, ankle clonus, and others.

In spastic dysarthria all aspects of articulation are impaired—respiration, phonation, and sound differentiation. Tongue and lip adjustments cannot be made with precision because of inadequate control, causing sound production to be inaccurate. In severe cases the individual is virtually speechless because he is only able to produce undifferentiated vocalizations that can scarcely be recognized as speech. In mild cases, the misarticulations sound like no more than a slight clumsiness or oral inaccuracy which has little or no effect on intelligibility.

Because of hypertonus and competing muscle contractions, the articulation rate is characteristically slower than normal and sounds labored or effortful. Adventitious sounds are often produced as the speaker struggles to carry out articulation movements. As would be expected, the normal rhythmic patterns of articulation are replaced by an irregular flow that lacks the fine changes in rate which help carry intellectual and emotional meanings. Sounds requiring adjustment of the front of the tongue are often particularly hard for the spastic. Tight jaw muscles are also common. Spastic dysarthria is aggravated by stress and tension, and reduced by relaxation. Articulation worsens as the speed and complexity of speech increases.

Comparable defects are heard in the vocal aspects of articulation. Fine inflectional changes in pitch are replaced by inappropriate pitch changes because of the effortful and uncoordinated movements of the laryngeal muscles. Vocal force is affected by laryngeal and respiratory incoordination, so that normal stress patterns are absent and abrupt explosive variations in force occur. Phonatory movements in the larynx are not properly synchronized with tongue and lip movement, so that voicing errors occur. Vocal quality may be "tight" and strained because of the excessive tensions in the larynx and in the muscles that adjust the resonators. Quite often the voice is intermittently hypernasal during connected speech. Some attempts have been made to ameliorate hypernasality by the same surgical procedures used to compensate for velar insufficiency in cleft palate.

Disordered breathing is often prominent. Vital capacity is typically reduced because respiratory movements are restricted, so that there is not enough air for the normal breath groupings of connected speech. Abdominal and thoracic movements are not in phase, as they should be in normal respiration. Inspiratory movements tend to be "jerky," and control of exhalation suffers from the same deficiencies that characterize other movements.

Dysarthria in Athetosis

Motor disorders in athetosis vary in detail but have in common involuntary and uncontrolled movements that interfere with coordination. These movements are sometimes slow and rhythmic or "worm-like," but they may also be irregular and quick, or explosive, or may even be of a flailing type, which disrupts arm and leg movement particularly. A prominent feature of athetosis is increase in involuntary motion under stress and tension. If the patient is thoroughly relaxed he may move normally, or nearly so, but under stress coordination is grossly defective. Often the athetoid speaker's involuntary facial grimaces, head movements, and inspiratory gasps signal that he is about to say something. Note that athetosis is a form of *secondary incoordination,* meaning that coordinations are disrupted only because accessory movements have been superimposed on what would otherwise have been normal actions.

There is considerable variability in articulation from one speaker to the next, but the individual characteristics in any given case should not be difficult to interpret if the basic nature of athetosis is kept in mind. The movements necessary to produce the prosodic features of speech are poorly executed, depending on the severity of the speaker's disorder. Athetoid and spastic dysarthria may sound very much alike because intelligibility is reduced in each disorder for similar reasons.

Dysarthria in Ataxia

The motor symptoms of *ataxia* are of a somewhat diverse character, but in general they are caused by a breakdown in the *primary* coordinating mechanisms of the central nervous system. These mechanisms include the proprioceptive input networks that provide the *cerebellar* circuits with information needed for the control of balance and movement. Disorders of posture, balance, and gait are prominent in ataxia. For instance, an ataxic patient who is asked to stand with his feet together and eyes closed will sway abnormally or even fall (positive *Romberg sign*). Ataxic gait is reeling and "drunken," with the legs spread to maintain balance. Because the patient cannot sense and control the direction and extent of muscle movement, his actions will be imprecise. For instance, if asked to point directly ahead with his eyes closed he will typically swing his arm beyond the midline ("past pointing"). Reciprocal or alternating movements are not performed smoothly because the patient cannot brake one motion properly in order to execute another. Muscle tone is reduced.

Ataxic dysarthria has several possible features. There may be marked oral inaccuracy and "mouthing" or mumbling of words. Articulation movements are not executed with normal force, causing weakness or loss of audibility. These characteristics are caused partly by the reduction in muscle tone. Because the patient cannot sense and control the direction and extent of movement, articulation adjustments will be imprecise and sluggish. In severe cases the patient may be unintelligible, or nearly so. Another dysarthric symptom is "scanning speech," so called because it bears a superficial resemblance to the way a poem might be read to bring out its metric structure. Actually, the patient speaks in a measured, monotonous, and uninflected manner because he cannot accomplish the fine variations in rate, force, and vocal melody that exist in normal speech. In contrast to monotonous or scanning speech some ataxic patients speak with inappropriate patterns of pitch, rate, and force, sometimes explosively, as in athetoid dysarthria.

Being a disorder of the major *synergic* center for movement, ataxia leaves a deficit that neither training nor treatment can reduce beyond a certain point. The situation is not entirely hopeless, however. Although the basic proprioceptive-motor loops are defective the speaker can use tactile, visual, and other sensory cues as substitutes for normal proprioceptive control. The training principles are, in fact, the same as those suggested for lower motor neuron dysarthria in which there is also an irreducible defect: self-monitoring, extensive perceptual training, drill on the sounds of speech, voluntary control of expressive movements, and the greatest possible level of motivation.

CENTRAL DYSARTHRIA

Although not new, the idea that there is a disorder of articulation that can be called central dysarthria is not found in clearly defined form in the speech pathology literature. Nevertheless, it seems to be the best conceptual basis on which to interpret systematically certain expressive disabilities and relate them to other neurogenic disorders of articulation. The basic concept is that central dysarthria consists of an inability to acquire or execute normally learned articulation movements, but without any muscular weakness or paralysis. This in part is what is conventionally meant by apraxia (sometimes *dyspraxia)*, but the definition is extended to include both acquired and developmental forms of the disorder. A central dysarthria of developmental origin, according to our paradigm, is a neurophysiologically based absence of the normal ability to lay down engrams for articulation. Patients with acquired central dysarthria have, in contrast, "forgotten" speech responses because of brain injury.

The generally recognized forms of speech apraxia, which we have equated with central dysarthria, are motor apraxia, ideomotor apraxia, and amnesic apraxia.

In *motor apraxia* (sometimes called *innervatory, limb-kinetic,* or *cortical apraxia*) there is slowing, awkwardness, stiffening, or clumsiness of motion, but the general pattern of action is carried out more or less correctly. Such a patient gives the impression of a mild weakness, paralysis, or defect of coordination, although the basic capacity for movement proves to be normal when tested. The patient understands the intended movement, but his attempts to carry it out are slow, awkward, and misdirected. He may do relatively well if he works slowly, but poorly if he tries to move at normal or accelerated speed. The more complex the action, the greater his difficulty.

Articulation is similar to that in other forms of dysarthria in which the basic power of motion is limited. The responses for producing the various speech sounds may be grossly correct, but they lack normal precision, and speech intelligently is proportionately reduced. Sounds that require more complex muscular adjustments are most markedly affected, and the speaker's difficulties are accentuated when he attempts connected speech or is asked to speed up his rate. A differential diagnosis between this and other forms of dysarthria is difficult to make with confidence, and a final decision must depend on general diagnostic findings, rather than on speech characteristics alone.

In *ideomotor* (*ideokinetic*) apraxia the patient is unable to execute movements voluntarily, even though he understands what is wanted and may be able to carry them out involuntarily. For instance, he cannot close his fist on request, but does so readily in grasping an object. Many of these brain-injured patients have difficulty moving the muscles of the face, tongue, lips, and jaw. When asked, they are unable to smile, open and close the mouth, move the tongue in various ways, or imitate simple speech sounds, but a patient who cannot imitate [p] will make essentially the same movements puffing on his pipe. Severe cases may seem wholly speechless and appear unable to initiate attempted speech responses; milder ones "stumble" on words. Unlike motor apraxia, the movements that can be made are carried out at normal speed.

In *amnesic* apraxia the patient seems to have forgotten the patterns of movement, although he can recognize and imitate the correct motions when they are performed for him. His motor difficulties are comparable to the language disorder of *amnesic aphasia* in which words cannot be recalled, but can be recognized and repeated. Even though the apractic patient imitates correctly he does not retain the ability to say the word for any appreciable length of time.

A patient with *ideational* apraxia has trouble performing a complex series of actions and appears not to understand the "meaning" of the act. Given a familiar article such as a toothbrush, he may try to use it inappropriately—to comb his hair, for instance. If given a cigaret and match, he may put the match in his mouth and try to strike the cigaret on the match box. Some confusions in articulation among brain-injured patients may be correlates of this disorder.

Problems in learning motor speech in neurologically impaired children have not yet been analyzed in enough detail for us to categorize them as we have the acquired central dysarthrias. This may never be possible since acquired neurogenic disorders can be limited to a specific function, but developmental disorders of the same origin are usually more generalized and affect all learning. Nevertheless, there are a few suggestive analogs. One sometimes observes a clumsiness in the articulation of neurologically impaired children that looks similar to motor apraxia. Unusually severe and persistent difficulties in phonetic learning often look similar to amnesic and ideational apraxia. Diagnostically, the greatest problem is to differentiate central dysarthria of developmental origin from the disorders associated with perceptual disabilities, for the misarticulations in these two conditions can resemble each other closely.

62   Many discussions of apraxia stem from the original contributions of
      Liepmann, whose work and that of others is summarized in some de-
      tail by Schlesinger (259). Alternative references would be Brain (35)
      or Nielsen (214).

❧❧❧

HABILITATION OR REHABILITATION IS THE ULTIMATE OBJECTIVE OF ALL study and research in speech pathology. The topics we have discussed up to this point have meaning only insofar as they contribute to this end. For practical reasons our treatment of diagnosis and training must be limited to a summary of principles. In the final analysis, however, only principles can be taught, for the successful practice of speech correction, although dependent on a thorough mastery of factual information, is an *art* which can be learned only through experience, an art that demands a high level of skill, insight, resourcefulness, and creative imagination.

This discussion must be limited to the correction of defective articulation, but in clinical practice articulation training is often inseparably related to language training. This applies particularly

7   *diagnosis and training*

to children with developmental delay, for they usually have needs in both areas. In a sense, phonetic skills are secondary to language, and when there are deficiencies in language, they must either take precedence in programming or receive primary emphasis. Improvement in articulation can be expected as an extra dividend in language training. The same principle holds for adults with foreign dialect and in some degree for older children with any kind of articulation disorder. More often than not, language instruction is the logical starting point in working with mentally retarded and neurologically impaired children.

PRINCIPLES OF DIAGNOSIS

Thorough and perceptive diagnosis is indispensable to successful training. If some of the observations that follow seem self-evident, remember that a significant proportion of all failures in speech correction can be traced to the neglect of elementary principles of diagnosis.

> 63   For a full treatment of diagnostic techniques and materials the reader is referred to a book in this series by Darley (65) and to Johnson, Darley, and Spriestersbach (148).

Clinical diagnosis has three objectives: (1) to *describe* the disorder as seen in each individual; (2) to *identify* and *analyze* the causes or conditions which are antecedent to it, or which cause it   **85** to persist; and (3) to *synthesize* all available information into a coherent picture of the total problem. All of these interrelated diagnostic steps are necessary before training can be planned intelligently. Diagnostic study must be adequate in breadth to make certain that no possible etological factor of any significance has been overlooked, and in depth to assure that the nature and extent of any deficits are understood as fully as possible.

Moreover, diagnosis must be thought of as a continuing process, not as a step to be completed before training and then forgotten. At best the information gathered before training can lead only to a tentative diagnosis, which is a base for initial treatment planning. The diagnostic hypotheses are then tested by applying the appropriate treatment and training measures. These, however, must be continuously evaluated as to their success or failure. Observing the person under treatment in this way will confirm or deny the tentative diagnosis and provide new insights. Only through such *diagnostic teaching* can the clinician hope to gain adequate understanding of the etiology in a given case. There is also no other way to appreciate the unique behavior and personality traits of the patient and the interaction among all these factors. Most really firm diagnoses are, in fact, to be made only in retrospect.

The *descriptive* part of diagnosis calls for a thorough and detailed study of the misarticulations in order to identify the speaking patterns that must be changed. The techniques are simple, but they require that the clinician have great personal skill in speech analysis—a skill he cannot acquire without sophisticated understanding of the structure and dynamics of spoken language. Articulation is analyzed by listening to samples of spontaneous speech in various systematic ways, and by preparing a *phonetic inventory*. To obtain this inventory various kinds of stimuli—pictures, toys, and printed material—are used as a means of getting the speaker to attempt words containing the sounds being tested. Methods of taking a phonetic inventory are described by Darley (65), who is a codesigner of one of the most detailed articulation tests. Another approach, which stresses the importance of testing sounds in all phonetic contexts, is suggested in a recent book by McDonald (180). The *Laradon Articulation Scale* (76), although not yet as widely used as some others, applies certain linguistic concepts to the analysis of articulation skills. Still other articulation tests, some of them available commercially, are listed in the bibliography at the end of this book (18, 19, 40, 54, 64, 104, 120, 133, 142, 203). Many clinicians prefer to develop their own testing materials. A phonetic inventory enables the examiner to locate the most obvious articulation errors in a limited speech sample, but further observation is necessary, since even the most thorough test misses errors that occur under some conditions.

64   Both Milisen (192) and Van Riper (318) discuss what they term *deep testing.*

The prosodic features of speech—rate, inflection, melody, and stress—must also be noted carefully since deficiencies in these can cause a conspicuous defect even though the sounds are otherwise produced correctly. Such widely different conditions as foreign dialect and cerebellar ataxia illustrate the point.

A thorough search for the possible causes of the disorder must be made, for they should be eliminated if possible or compensated for if they cannot be eliminated. Even in apparently simple cases an adequate diagnosis often requires highly specialized examinations. The minimum schedule for all cases normally includes: (1) a careful medical, developmental, and social case history; (2) an examination of the orofacial structure and an appraisal of the functional integrity of the articulation musculature; (3) the measurement of hearing and, in some cases, other senses; (4) an assessment of learning abilities and disabilities; (5) an evaluation of educational achievement if the patient is in school or, if not, of his vocational adjustment; and (6) an exploration, in appropriate depth, of his behavior, personality, and social and emotional adjustment. The information gathered in these categories is then used to determine the necessity for additional medical, dental, psychological, or other kinds of examination. How far the diagnostic study should be carried is a matter of judgment, but no diagnosis can be considered complete unless one feels with reasonable confidence that no factor of possible etiological significance has been overlooked.

After all the pertinent information has been gathered, the pieces of the puzzle must be put together in order to develop an initial treatment and training plan. It is critical to remember that rarely, if ever, will an articulation disorder have a single cause. Therefore all possible etiological factors must be identified, the contribution of each evaluated, and a decision made on the implications this information has for treatment planning. It is equally important to recognize that the individual's own unique traits of behavior and personality determine the way these causative factors exert their influence. Recognizing that fact is one of the keys to successful training; there is no standard educational prescription for any kind of articulation disorder.

Some comments should be made about the *team approach* to diagnosis. With few exceptions, thorough diagnosis calls for more than one specialist; the speech pathologist, audiologist, psychologist, social worker, and various medical and dental specialists are among those regularly needed. Our information about handicapping conditions, although still deficient in many respects, has become so extensive that no single person can have all the knowledge needed in a comprehensive diagnosis. The cleft-palate team is an excellent illustration of the point: here the minimum team includes a social worker, plastic surgeon, otologist, orthodontist, prosthodontist, and speech pathologist. Other specialists, for example a psychologist, are needed for an ideal team. Such an elaborate array is not always required, but there are few individuals with defective speech who will not benefit if their problems are explored by specialists other than the speech pathologist. Failure to utilize all possible resources for help is a serious clinical error.

The best arrangement for multidisciplinary or interdisciplinary management is one in which the various specialists first make their individual examinations then meet in a staffing session to exchange information and arrive at joint diagnostic conclusions and recommendations for treatment. This has become standard practice in larger centers, but a speech pathologist working in a small community or in a public school may feel that such a procedure is too elaborate for him. This may be true up to a point, and it might be better if he referred some of his cases to larger centers. He should never do so, however, without careful consideration, for the number of such cases may be fewer than he realizes. There are few communities so small that they do not contain people with the information and skills needed to handle most cases. A speech pathologist, the child's physician, his teacher, the school psychologist. and the school principal can make an excellent team—one which, in fact, because it is on the scene can be far more effective than a group of highly trained specialists in a neighboring city.

ARTICULATION TRAINING: GENERAL CONSIDERATIONS

Case Finding and Selection

Locating the children and adults who need articulation training is no particular problem in a community speech and hearing center or rehabilitation center, since people with communication disorders seek out such agencies or are referred to them. In other situations, particularly in the public schools, case finding is an important responsibility of the speech pathologist.

A *screening survey* to identify children with defective speech is the usual starting point. If the speech correction program is being organized for the first time, the entire school population should be screened; otherwise, only the children who are entering the school for the first time need to be examined. The registration procedures carried out by the school principal or whoever receives the child should include questions about special services the child has received (or needed) in his former school or, if this is his first year, whether or not he is thought to have speech or other disabilities that might affect his learning and school adjustment. Systematic procedures should be set up for recording such information in the child's school folder, and for reporting suspected speech problems to the person in charge of speech correction services.

There are a number of simple but effective ways in which large school populations can be screened quickly and reliably. If the number of pupils is not too large it is preferable for the examiner to observe each one individually under conditions where he can listen to a brief but adequate speech sample. If the number to be screened is too large for this procedure, an alternative method—which many speech pathologists prefer in any event—is to place the primary responsibility for finding children who may need speech services on the classroom teacher.

In this case the classroom teacher is asked to be alert to any speech peculiarities in her children, and a plan is set up for reporting their names to the speech correctionist. This can be a satisfactory way of finding children who should be given individual examinations. Teachers are not, of course, expected to know what is wrong with the child's speech (although their descriptions often provide valuable diagnostic clues); they are asked simply to report any child they think might have a speech problem. One must have established good relationships with the teachers and have helped them learn what to listen and watch for, but this can usually be accomplished without too much difficulty by explanations at teachers' meetings, by printed instructions, and in other ways.

This method will bring in many children who do not have significant speech problems, but if the teachers are cooperative and informed, not many children who do have problems will be overlooked—particularly if the teachers are encouraged to make later referrals if they notice a speech peculiarity that was missed on the first round. After this initial screening, each child must be diagnosed in whatever depth seems indicated. Many will be eliminated after examination by the speech correctionist; the remainder should go through whatever diagnostic procedures have been decided on. In addition to the general screening, there should also be a systematic recheck of the children who have been dismissed from speech training, since relapses are unfortunately common.

Next, cases most in need of remedial training must be selected. Regrettably, there are few situations where the supply of services is fully equal to the demand; on the contrary, most speech correctionists, in public schools and elsewhere, have a larger potential case load than they can possibly assume, and some difficult decisions must be made. Under the pressure of such a situation, some try to divide their time among too many children, with the disappointing results that inevitably follow insufficient treatment. There is no invariable rule for an efficient case load size since the nature of the cases and the way in which they are handled make a difference, but 50 is probably the limit for typical public school programs where children are seen twice weekly in small groups. Not only must each case have sufficiently intensive training to progress, if he can, but to do an acceptable job the correctionist should reserve enough time for record keeping, parent and teacher conferences, and other indispensable collateral duties. Any other course of action is wasteful and inefficient, no matter how impressive the statistics in the annual report on the number of cases "served" may appear.

A comprehensive list of the factors to be weighed and balanced in choosing cases would be difficult to draw up. Among the important considerations, however, are the severity of the defect and the extent to which it impairs communication, the degree to which it is a source of stress for the individual (and his family and associates in some cases), the probability of success, the likelihood of improvement through maturation, and age. Other things being equal, early training is much to be preferred, even though there is some hope that the child will "outgrow" his defect. Once a

65   For a discussion of some of the factors which seem to have value in
      predicting improvement through maturation, see Carter and Buck (54)
      and other titles listed at the end of their article.

training program has been started, it should be continued until the individual has achieved the goals that were set for him. Finally, one should not forget those cases who were not selected for training, since the reasons why they were not taken can change rapidly.

Programming

When an adequate tentative diagnosis has been made, the next consideration is programming. The development of a total program of management must be thought through with the utmost care before actual training is begun. The program must provide a comprehensive *treatment plan* which will meet as nearly as possible all the individual's needs that have been crystallized by diagnosis, and the strategy for putting the treatment plan into effect must be planned. There must be a clear and specific definition of goals, both immediate and long-range, at which the remedial program is aimed.

Goal setting

All too often the correctionist begins a training program without a clear formulation of objectives. The ultimate goal in all cases is the best level of function the patient can be expected to achieve, but this must be defined in specific terms. In some cases the goal is completely normal communication; in others, it may have to be more limited. When irreversible factors, such as profound central nervous system pathology, limit the patient's potential, they must be faced realistically and the training objectives realistically defined. One whose attitudes are thoroughly professional will be as keenly interested in a person who can make only limited progress as he will in another who may become normal and is easy to work with. The key question is, "Can something, no matter how little, be done to help him function more adequately. and therefore live more happily and successfully?" Whatever the long-range goal, it should be broken down into a succession of subgoals, with particular thought given to the order in which the various phases of treatment should take place.

The treatment plan

One principle that cannot be emphasized too strongly is that a treatment plan must be *prescriptive,* that is, it should be tailored precisely to the needs of the individual. This may seem self-evident, but its neglect is a common error in the management of articulation disorders. Obviously not all articulation disorders that sound the same have the same cause. Even if they did, each child is unique and has his own ways of thinking, feeling, and behaving. This implies that the training techniques should be chosen with care. Many times a speech correctionist becomes enthusiastic about a particular method, or has learned only one, and adheres sedulously to it. But there is no single method that works best with all cases, and the skilled practitioner is resourceful in adapting methods to needs.

Most clinical treatment is based on a philosophy of "total push," that is, an attempt to deal with every possible factor that may be contributing to the individual's failure to function up to the level of his full potential. The wisdom of such an approach is obvious. A typical child with defective articulation might, for instance, be doing poorly in school, have health problems, be meeting so much rejection from his schoolmates that he has become disturbed and unhappy, and be a source of such anxiety to his parents that life at home is full of stress for the whole family. Articulation training alone would be ineffective. A better plan would take care of his health needs, take steps to improve his school success, ameliorate his social and emotional problems, *and* improve his articulation.

Moreover, these different kinds of help must be put together carefully in such a way that each part of the treatment plan fits with the others into an effective "total push." The only way this can really be accomplished is by group conference, the team approach, in which all the specialists who will administer services work together. Time-consuming as this may be, any other procedure wastes more time than it saves.

Anything that can be done to eliminate the cause of defective articulation has first priority. If an orofacial defect is found to be an etiology, speech training should be deferred until surgical or dental treatment has reached a predetermined stage. For example, if velar insufficiency is diagnosed as the major cause of a cleft-palate child's speech deviations, then plastic surgery, not speech training, obviously comes first. The same would hold for orthodontia if a dental malocclusion is felt to be a factor. Application of this general rule must be tempered with judgment, of course. It might be that some phases of the defect could be attacked after palate surgery, but others will have to wait until orthodontia is completed later. There may also be misarticulations not directly associated with structural deviations, along with some that are. In this case the functional errors can probably receive attention at once. Young preschool and primary grade children may need speech and language stimulation even though they have dysglossic errors that cannot be corrected. Not rarely therapy is given simply for its *supportive* value, and there are many other similar contingencies.

When structural deviations cannot be treated successfully, or if there is some reason why measures such as surgery or orthodontia are not likely to be carried out, the speaker can often be taught compensatory movements for production of the speech sounds that give him trouble. Briefly, this involves articulation of the error sounds by nonstandard movements which nevertheless produce the desired acoustic results. A person with marked prognathism, for instance, may be unable to produce an acceptable [s] in the standard manner, but he can usually learn tongue adjustments that channel the breath in such a way as to circumvent his dental deformity. In some

66   A full account of methods by which compensatory movements can be taught is given by Van Riper (319).

cases defective speech is the only reason why surgical or dental treatment is considered, the individual's appearance and other function being satisfactory. After all factors are weighed the most practical decision may be to teach compensatory movements. Unless there are good reasons to the contrary, however, most speech pathologists prefer restoration of the physical structure. At best, good speech is more difficult to produce in nonstandard ways, for phonetic theory teaches that economy of effort is one of the reasons why speech sounds are produced as they are. Dental or surgical treatment must usually be followed by speech training, since previously existing habits will tend to persist.

Coordinating the articulation training with other parts of the treatment plan is not usually difficult. In a school setting, the speech correctionist should keep in constant touch with the classroom teacher, and with any other people who are working with the child, to make certain that their programs are mutually supportive. At any given time emphasis should be placed on activities that will make the greatest contribution to the "total push." For example, it might be best if speech training yielded to remedial reading at some point in the interests of better school progress. Or a child may go "stale" on articulation training and benefit from a period of rest. The role of articulation training for children who are receiving psychotherapy for significant emotional problems sometimes needs careful consideration, for there may be interference. One should remember, however, that if an individual's speech is a source of stress, one of the most sensible measures is to help him talk better. In any event, all such questions are to be answered by free communication among the members of the team.

The therapy setting

Conventionally, individual training has been preferred, on the assumption that it leads to the most rapid progress. Many correctionists handle cases in groups only because it enables them to assume a larger case load. Individual training is undoubtedly best for some cases because it does allow intensive help which is impossible in a group.

But there is no general rule, and group therapy has certain advantages that should not be overlooked. Backus and Beasley (14) argue that, since speech is a communicative function, growth in articulation skills will proceed more quickly and surely in a social situation. Their line of reasoning is persuasive, and the specific techniques they propose seem particularly effective in providing a psychological climate for socializing and motivating activities. Even if this approach is not followed in its entirety, the interpersonal reactions of a group situation can still be used to create a favorable setting for articulation improvement. A combination of individual and group training is an obvious compromise, with the individual sessions devoted to activities that are not needed by the majority of the group.

ARTICULATION TRAINING: METHODS AND PROCEDURES

Training the Receptive Processes

Typical individuals with defective articulation are unaware that their speech is considered defective or "different" by listeners. We pay little conscious attention to the fine details of our own articulation; instead, we attend primarily to what we want to say and depend upon automatic mechanisms for the execution of the speech movements. Nevertheless, if a normal speaker misarticulates a word or suffers a slip of the tongue he will ordinarily correct his error—quite automatically in most cases. He does so because the articulation lapse has triggered an alarm in the input-output loop for speech control. This does not happen in the speaker whose articulation is defective, except in special cases. Because of faulty learning and habituation, his input-output circuits accept a misarticulation as correct. It is therefore easy to understand why even an intelligent adult with good hearing may not realize that he has a severe lisp, or why a child, admonished for an [r] substitution, may protest, "I *said* wabbit!" Training in speech reception is a necessary antecedent to the establishment of new and correct motor responses.

Some people with articulation disorders may have become aware that they do not speak correctly, either through self-observation or because they have been told. Even so, they are still unlikely to know exactly *how* their articulation differs, again because they listen to the content, not the form, of their utterances. Articulation errors that they detect readily in others (or in their own recorded speech) pass unrecognized in their own speech. Because of these characteristics of the speaking and speech-learning process, perceptual training is an important role in the correction of defective articulation, and is the usual starting point in a remedial program.

A primary purpose of perceptual training is to teach the individual with defective speech to attend specifically to his own speech signals, and to compare what he hears with "memories" or percepts he has built up through training. What this training develops is an internal *comparator* mechanism which will be used later, when he is trying to develop new neuromuscular patterns for correct articulation. In the beginning he will not pay conscious attention to feedback information, so that a new listening and feeling set must be established—a step that is not necessarily easy. Because he accepts his defective speech as correct, he must learn to listen perceptively to his own speech in order to recognize its fine details and compare them with the kind of speech he is trying to develop.

Through the influence of Van Riper (319) the procedure through which these goals can be reached has come to be referred to as *ear training*. This term may be too narrow, since the feedback cues that should be exploited include touch and kinesthesia as well as audition; nevertheless, the techniques he suggests form the basis for a practical program to teach perceptual skills, and are recommended. The methods are grouped into four categories: (1) *isolation;* (2) *stimulation;* (3) *identification,* and (4) *discrimination.*

The method of isolation is based on the theory that one cannot acquire the necessary perceptual skills readily if the sounds to which he should attend are embedded in the complex patterns of ongoing speech or even, at the start, in single words. He is therefore taught, through a phonic approach, that words can be broken down into syllables and sounds as separable acoustic units of speech. An untrained child who says "wabbit" cannot be expected to realize that the word can be analyzed into sound "families" and then put together again; he perceives words, phrases, and possibly even longer linguistic configurations as wholes. Before developing new expressive movements he must first learn to recognize the smaller perceptual units of the individual speech sounds. Incidentally, do not be troubled by the fact that many of the phonemes of English cannot be produced in isolation, for one can learn to recognize individual sounds even though they must be spoken as parts of syllables in the course of listening drills. All of the *continuant* sounds [s], [z], [ʃ], [ʒ], [θ], [ð], [f], [v], [m], [n] can, for purposes of perceptual training, be produced in isolation. The rest of the nonsyllabic sounds are best presented as parts of syllables. Before perceptual training is successfully completed, one must be able to detect with confidence the individual sounds as they occur in the context of complex speech.

The method of *stimulation* emphasizes that extensive, varied, and rich listening experiences are indispensable to successful perceptual training. Some cases learn phonic analysis easily, and others progress slowly; but neither the speech correctionist nor the patient should allow impatience to cause them to move to the next step before listening skills are perfected through adequate stimulation.

Identification enables one to recognize each of the speech sounds and to become aware of its unique characteristics. For example, the patient is taught to recognize that there *is* an [s] sound and to identify its distinctive sibilant quality. Sensory cues other than hearing should be used as much as possible throughout perceptual training, for this kind of input information is of great importance in normal feedback loops. Learning is therefore most efficient if kinesthetic and tactual cues for the sound are associated with auditory cues. Although not a part of the normal input information for articulation, visual cues may be of supplementary help.

The ability to *discriminate* requires that one sound can be distinguished from all others, but the most critical distinctions are those between error sounds and correct ones. If a child substitutes [θ] for [s], for example, he must learn to pay particular attention to the difference between them so that later he can tell whether or not he has articulated a good [s]. If the error sound is nonstandard, as in the case of a lateral lisp, the same careful techniques must be followed for discrimination between correct and incorrect responses.

plex sound configurations, there is probably a better chance of learning the correct articulation of words. It is best to start with words that have simpler configurations of sounds and less difficult articulations—monosyllables without consonant blends—and systematically expand to longer words and more intricate phonetic contexts. The speaker's *self-monitoring set* is most important. Early in the training program he must learn to be conscious of the way he talks and be willing to make an effort toward conscious control; there is no alternate route. Throughout the entire training process he learns monitoring attitudes and skills, but these cannot be fully used without the strongest possible *motivation*.

72   An extensive discussion of teaching devices for the transfer of new responses to speech will be found in Van Riper (319).

Muscle training

Exercises to strengthen and activate the articulation muscles and improve coordination are indispensable to the treatment of certain disorders of articulation. With cerebral-palsied children, for instance, the speech pathologist must focus on exercises that develop neuromuscular potentials just as the physical therapist prepares a child to learn to walk by special methods of exercise. In the same way, the muscles of the palatopharyngeal valving mechanism must be activated and strengthened as a standard part of the postoperative training for cleft-palate speakers.

There are some who feel that muscle training *per se* is not particularly valuable except in special cases such as those just mentioned. This view, however, should not be accepted too quickly, nor should the effects of tongue, lip, jaw, and breathing exercises be underestimated, even when the articulation disorder is judged to be primarily functional. These exercises need not be administered routinely, and judgment must be used. Nevertheless, it is entirely possible that such exercises, properly subordinated to the larger objectives of the training program, will contribute to articulation improvement in most cases. Research is inadequate, but there are reasons to suspect that a significant physiological *anlage* may underlie articulation dysfunction more often than is generally recognized. At any rate, this working hypothesis is recommended in the treatment of articulation disorders.

73   Probably the best source of muscle training exercises is one of the texts on speech training for cerebral-palsied children, such as Cass (56), Meacham (188), or Rutherford (249). The "chewing" techniques of Froeschels (93) are also of great interest in this connection.

Lesson plans and therapy materials

The organization of lesson plans and the selection of teaching materials are matters of considerable practical importance. With respect to planning each therapy session it should suffice to say that there must *be* a plan, written or not, in which the objectives for the day are thoughtfully considered, clearly defined, and properly related to the total therapy plan that should have been worked out before training was begun. Materials selected for therapy sessions should meet certain criteria: (1) they should sustain interest and attention, and in this sense be enjoyable; (2) they should involve activities that contribute directly to the objectives of the therapy session; and (3) insofar as possible they should be worth doing in themselves as a learning experience. Materials for training sessions with adults are not so hard to develop, since the problems of sustaining attention are not so great as they are with children; remote goals are easier for the adult to appreciate.

Materials are more important with children, however, although the child should never become so engrossed in the activity itself (beating the teacher at word lotto!) that he loses sight of why he is having speech lessons. The speech correction literature is so full of descriptions of teaching materials and separate books on the subject that we shall not even try to offer references. One would do well, however, to evaluate many of the speech correction "games" in light of the criteria outlined above.

The preparation of a speech correctionist who expects to work with children should make him familiar with their learning processes and with the methods and materials suitable for different age levels. Students who resist courses in professional education and teaching methods should realize that the best materials for articulation training have much in common with those used for reading readiness, reading (and remedial reading), and other language arts instruction. And finally, there is no substitute for creative imagination in planning teaching activities of any kind.

Habituating the New Response

The final step in articulation training aims to bring the individual to the point where he functions as a normal individual, with an ability to communicate in accordance with his needs. Hopefully, the old habit patterns will be replaced by correct neuromuscular responses operating under newly established automatic control mechanisms. In many cases this goal can be fully reached, although sometimes only after a long period of habituation. In others, unfortunately, it may always be necessary for the speaker to exercise some conscious control over the way he talks in order to avoid conspicuous and embarrassing misarticulations. The child with cerebral palsy, for example, must always exercise this control, for he can never be expected to walk, talk, or carry out any other motor activity without conscious attention to what he is doing. There are also some individuals whose speech disorders seem to be functional, but who cannot achieve fully habituated normal articulation. The necessity for self-monitoring may perhaps be regrettable, yet it is a fact of life and should be accepted as such.

Although there are no unusual learning principles involved in the habituation of new speech responses, certain major points should be mentioned. First, a speaker can never trust habit to give him normal articulation unless he has passed through a period during which he was willing and able to pay conscious attention to to the sound of his own speech. It is easy for even a young child to understand that he must pay attention so that he can talk a certain way; the problem is to keep him motivated and reminded. There is, of course, no stronger force than approval and success in communication. If incorrect responses are approved and successful, the consequence is inevitable. The transfer of training activities must therefore be planned with these ideas in mind.

It is quite unrealistic to ask either a child or an adult to monitor carefully every word he speaks. Consequently, the responses to be habituated should be limited to certain sounds or a core vocabulary until habituation is accomplished and new sounds and words can be introduced. Perhaps monitoring can be confined to certain "good speech" situations at first, then systematically broadened. Thus a child who had infantile speech but now knows how to produce [θ] might be given a list of common "th-words" which he is to watch for and attempt to use in certain situations, for example, at the dinner table, during certain school periods (such as "show and tell," or reading aloud), or at other times that seem appropriate. With children, the cooperation of the parents and teachers will contribute greatly to the success of a transfer and habituation program. If they are to be good helpers, they must be fully informed on what has been planned and the methods they should use to reinforce the child's correct speech attempts. The resourceful speech correctionist should be able to invent many original mnemonic devices to help the individual remember self-monitoring.

74   See Lillywhite's article, "Make Mother a Clinician" (167).

A review of earlier activities such as perceptual training, strengthening drill, and the practice of new responses in contextual speech will reinforce measures to habituate good articulation. One can expect great differences in the speed with which different individuals come to use their new responses habitually, depending on motivation and many other factors, some unknown. At best this step probably takes longer than any other in the total articulation training program. Neither the patient nor the speech correctionist should become discouraged if progress seems slow. There is inevitably a period during which new speech habits break down under stress or pressure. If relapses occur—and this is always a risk—the possible causes should be sought. These are commonly incomplete training, poor motivation, and emotional interference. Appropriate measures will be suggested by the nature of the unfavorable influence. If it turns out that the speaker is one who must always monitor with more than the normal degree of care, then the problem of motivating him to do so must be faced.

bibliography

1. Abt, I. A., H. M. Adler, and P. Bartelme, "The Relationship Between the Onset of Speech and Intelligence," *Journal of the American Medical Association*, XCIII (1929).
2. Ainsworth, S., *Galloping Sounds* (Magnolia, Mass.: Expression Co., 1946).
3. _____, *Speech Correction Methods* (Englewood Cliffs, N.J.: Prentice-Hall, Inc., 1948).
4. Albright, R. W., "The Motor Abilities of Speakers with Good and Poor Articulation," *Speech Monographs*, XV (1948), 164-72.
5. Allen, Evelyn Y., Martha E. Black, Marjorie Burkland, Margaret C. Byrne, Mary S. Farquhar, Esther L. Herbert, and Mary Lu Robertson, "Case Selection in the Public Schools," *Journal of Speech and Hearing Disorders*, XXXI (1966), 157-60.
6. Allport, Floyd, *Social Psychology* (New York: Houghton-Mifflin Co., 1924).
7. Ammons, R. B., and Helen S. Ammons, *The Full-Range Picture Vocabulary Test* (Missoula, Montana: Psychological Test Specialists, 1948).
8. Anders, Q. M., "A Study of the Personal and Social Adjustment of Children with Functional Articulation Defects." Unpublished Ph.D. dissertation, University of Wisconsin, 1945.
9. Anderson, V. A., "Auditory Memory Span as Tested by Speech Sounds," *American Journal of Psychology*, LII (1939), 95-99.
10. _____, *Improving the Child's Speech* (New York: Oxford University Press, 1953).
11. Aungst, Lester F., and James V. Frick, "Auditory Discrimination Ability and Consistency of Articulation of /r/," *Journal of Speech and Hearing Disorders*, XXVIII (1964), 76-85.
12. Backus, Ollie L., "Group Structure in Speech Therapy," in *Handbook*

of Speech Pathology, ed. L. E. Travis (New York: Appleton-Century-Crofts, Inc., 1957).

13. ———, "Speech Rehabilitation Following Excision of the Tip of the Tongue," *American Journal of Diseases of Children,* LX (1940).

14. ——— and J. Beasley, *Speech Therapy with Children* (New York: Houghton-Mifflin Co., 1951).

15. ——— and H. M. Dunn, "Use of Conversation Patterns to Promote Speed and Retention of Learning," *Journal of Speech Disorders,* XII (1947), 135-42.

16. Bangs, J. L., "A Clinical Analysis of the Articulatory Defects of the Feeble Minded," *Journal of Speech Disorders,* VII (1942), 343-56.

17. Bangs, Tina E., "Evaluating Children with Language Delay," *Journal of Speech and Hearing Disorders,* XXVI (1961).

18. Barker, Janet O., "A Numerical Measure of Articulation," *Journal of Speech and Hearing Disorders,* XXV (1960).

19. ——— and G. England, "A Numerical Measure of Articulation: Further Developments," *Journal of Speech and Hearing Disorders,* XXVII (1962).

20. Barrows, S. T., and K. H. Hall, *Games and Jingles for Speech Development* (Magnolia, Mass.: Expression Co., 1936).

21. Bateman, Barbara, and Janis Wetherell, "Psycholinguistic Aspects of Mental Retardation," *Mental Retardation,* III (1965), 8-13.

22. Beasley, J., "Group Therapy in the Field of Speech Correction," *Journal of the Exceptional Child,* XVII (1950), 102-7.

23. Beebe, H. H., "Auditory Memory Span for Meaningless Syllables," *Journal of Speech Disorders,* IX (1944), 273-75.

24. Bell, Dorothy, and Anita Hale, "Observations of Tongue-Thrust Swallow in Preschool Children," *Journal of Speech and Hearing Disorders,* XXVIII (1963), 195-97.

25. Bender, J. F., and V. M. Kleinfeld, *Principles and Practices of Speech Correction* (New York: Pitman Publishing Corp., 1938).

26. Berry, Mildred F., and Jon Eisenson, *Speech Disorders: Principles and Practices of Therapy* (New York: Appleton-Century-Crofts, Inc., 1956).

27. Bilto, E. W., "A Comparative Study of Certain Physical Abilities of Children with Speech Defects and Children with Normal Speech," *Journal of Speech Disorders,* VI (1941), 187-206.

28. Black, J. W., "The Pressure Component in the Production of Consonants," *Journal of Speech and Hearing Disorders,* XV (1950), 207-10.

29. Black, Martha E., *Speech Correction in the Schools* (Englewood Cliffs, N.J.: Prentice-Hall, Inc., 1964).

30. Blanton, M. G., and S. Blanton, *Speech Training for Children* (New York: Appleton-Century-Crofts, Inc., 1920).

31. Blattner, H., "An Experimental Study of the Testing of Pronunciation," *Speech Monographs,* XV (1948), 181-87.

32. Blomquist, B., "Diadochokinetic Movements of Nine-, Ten-, and Eleven-Year-Old Children," *Journal of Speech and Hearing Disorders,* XV (1950), 159-64.

33. Bloomer, H. Harlan, "Speech Defects Associated with Dental Abnormalities and Malocclusions," in *Handbook of Speech Pathology,* ed. L. E. Travis (New York: Appleton-Century-Crofts, Inc., 1957).

34. Bosma, James F., *Symposium on Oral Sensation and Perception* (Springfield, Ill.: Charles C Thomas, 1967).
35. Brain, Sir Russell, *Speech Disorders* (Washington, D.C.: Butterworth, Inc., 1961).
36. Brissey, F. L., and W. D. Trotter, "Social Relationships among Speech Defective Children," *Journal of Speech and Hearing Disorders,* XX (1955), 277-83.
37. Brodbeck, A. J., and O. C. Irwin, "The Speech Behavior of Infants Without Families," *Child Development,* XVII (1946).
38. Brookshire, Robert H., "Speech Pathology and the Experimental Analysis of Behavior," *Journal of Speech and Hearing Disorders,* XXXII (1967), 215-27.
39. Brown, F. W., "Baby Talkers," *Proceedings of American Speech Correction Association,* VI (1939), 127-42.
40. Bryngelson, B., and Esther Glaspey, *Speech in the Classroom* (with *Speech Improvement Cards*), 3rd Ed. (Chicago: Scott, Foresman & Co., 1962).
41. Burt, C., *The Backward Child* (New York: Appleton-Century-Crofts, Inc., 1937).
42. Byrne, Margaret, *The Child Speaks: A Speech Improvement Program for Kindergarten and First Grade* (New York: Harper and Row, Publishers, 1965).
43. Canter, Gerald J., "Speech Characteristics of Patients with Parkinson's Disease: I. Intensity, Pitch, and Duration," *Journal of Speech and Hearing Disorders,* XXVIII (1963), 221-29.
44. _____, "Speech Characteristics of Patients with Parkinson's Disease: II. Physiological Support for Speech," *Journal of Speech and Hearing Disorders,* XXX (1965), 44-49.
45. _____, "Speech Characteristics of Patients with Parkinson's Disease: III. Articulation, Diadochokinesis, and Over-All Speech Adequacy," *Journal of Speech and Hearing Disorders,* XXX (1965), 217-24.
46. Carhart, R., "Hearing Deficiencies and Speech Problems," *Journal of Speech Disorders,* VIII (1943), 247-56.
47. Carrell, James, "A Comparative Study of Speech Defective Children," Archives of Speech, I (1936), 179-203.
48. _____, "The Etiology of Sound Substitution Defects," *Speech Monographs,* IV (1937), 17-37.
49. _____ and Bangs, J. L., "Disorders of Speech Comprehension Associated with Language Retardation," *Nervous Child,* IX (1952), 64-76.
50. _____ and Tiffany, William R., *Phonetics: Theory and Application to Speech Improvement* (New York: McGraw-Hill Book Co., Inc., 1960).
51. Carroll, J. B., "Language Development," in *Encyclopedia of Educational Research,* 3rd Ed., ed. C. W. Harris (New York: The Macmillan Co., 1960).
52. _____, "Language Development in Children," in *Psycholinguistics,* ed. S. Saporta (New York: Holt, Rinehart & Winston, Inc., 1961).
53. Carrow, Sister Mary Arthur, "Linguistic Functioning of Bilingual and Monolingual Children," *Journal of Speech and Hearing Disorders,* XXII (1957).

54. Carter, E. T., and McKenzie W. Buck, "Prognostic Testing for Articulation Disorders among Children in the First Grade," *Journal of Speech and Hearing Disorders,* XXIII (1958).

55. Carterette, Edward C., ed., *Brain Function, Vol. 3: Speech, Language and Communication* (Berkeley: University of California Press, 1966).

56. Cass, M. T., *Speech Habilitation in Cerebral Palsy* (New York: Columbia University Press, 1951).

57. Chaiklin, Joseph, and Ira Ventry, "Functional Hearing Loss," in *Modern Developments in Audiology,* ed. James Jerger (New York: Academic Press, 1963).

58. Chreist, Fred M., *Foreign Accent* (Englewood Cliffs, N.J.: Prentice-Hall, Inc., 1964).

59. Cochran, L., "A New Phonetic Discrimination Test Using Words as Stimuli," *Speech Abstracts,* IV (1944), 37-42.

60. Cohen, Julian H., and Charles F. Hiehl, "Relation of Speech-Sound Discrimination Ability to Articulation-Type Speech Defects," *Journal of Speech and Hearing Disorders,* XXVIII (1963), 187-90.

61. Crickmay, Marie C., *Speech Therapy and the Bobath Approach to Cerebral Palsy* (Springfield, Ill.: Charles C Thomas, 1966).

62. Critchley, M., "Articulatory Defects in Aphasia," *Journal of Laryngology and Otology,* LXVI (1952).

63. Cruikshank, W. G., *et al., Perception and Cerebral Palsy* (Syracuse, N.Y.: Syracuse University Press, 1957).

64. Curry, E. T., L. Kennedy, L. Wagner, and W. Wilke, "A Phonographic Scale for the Measurement of Defective Articulation," *Journal of Speech Disorders,* VIII (1943), 123-26.

65. Darley, F. L., *Diagnosis and Appraisal of Communication Disorders* (Englewood Cliffs, N.J.: Prentice-Hall, 1964).

66. _____, "Speech Problems in the Aging," *Postgraduate Medicine,* XXXIII (1963).

67. Davis, E. A., "The Development of Linguistic Skill in Twins, Singletons with Siblings, and Only Children from Age Five to Ten Years," *University of Minnesota Child Welfare Monograph Series,* No. 14 (1937).

68. Davis, Hallowell, and S. Richard Silverman, *Hearing and Deafness,* Rev. Ed. (New York: Holt, Rinehart & Winston, Inc., 1963).

69. Dawson, L. O., "A Study of the Development of the Role of Articulation," *Elementary School Journal,* XXIX (1929), 610-15.

70. Day, Ella J., "The Development of Language in Twins, I. A Comparison of Twins and Single Children," *Child Development,* III (1932).

71. Di Carlo, Louis M., *The Deaf* (Englewood Cliffs, N.J.: Prentice-Hall, Inc., 1964).

72. Draegert, G. L., "Intelligibility Related to Articulation," *Speech Monographs,* XIII (1946), 50.

73. Dub, A., "Great Psychological Effects of the Minor Speech Defect," *Journal of Speech and Hearing Disorders,* XIII (1948), 251-58.

74. Dunn, L. M., *Peabody Picture Vocabulary Test* (Nashville, Tenn.: American Guidance Service, 1959).

75. _____ and J. O. Smith, *Peabody Language Development Kit* (Minneapolis, Minn.: American Guidance Service, 1963).

76. Edmonston, W., *The Laradon Articulation Scale* (Denver, Colo.: Laradon Hall, 1960).

77. Eisenson, Jon, Jeffery Auer, and John V. Irwin, *The Psychology of Communication* (New York: Appleton-Century-Crofts, Inc., 1963).

78. Elliott, J. C., "Personality Traits of School Children with Speech Deviations as Indicated by the California Test of Personality," *Speech Monographs,* XIX (1952), 158.

79. Engel, Dean C., Stanley Brandriet, Karen Erickson, K. Dale Gronhovd, and Gerald Gunderson, "Carryover," *Journal of Speech and Hearing Disorders,* XXXI (1966), 227-33.

80. Everhart, R. W., "The Relationships Between Articulation and Other Developmental Factors in Children," *Journal of Speech and Hearing Disorders,* XVIII (1953), 332-38.

81. Ewing, A. W. G., ed., *Educational Guidance and the Deaf Child* (Manchester, England: Manchester University Press, 1957).

82. Fairbanks, G., "Systematic Research in Experimental Phonetics: 1. A Theory of the Speech Mechanism as a Servosystem," *Journal of Speech and Hearing Disorders,* XIX (1954), 133-39.

83. _____, *Voice and Articulation Drillbook* (New York: Harper & Row, Publishers, 1940).

84. _____ and B. Bebout, "A Study of Minor Organic Deviations in Functional Disorders of Articulation: The Tongue," *Journal of Speech and Hearing Disorders,* XV (1950), 248-352.

85. _____ and Evelyn Green, "A Study of Minor Organic Deviations in Functional Disorders of Articulation: 2. Dimensions and Relationships of the Lips," *Journal of Speech and Hearing Disorders,* XV (1950), 165-68.

86. _____ and M. V. H. Lintner, "A Study of Minor Organic Deviations in Functional Disorders of Articulation: The Teeth and Hard Palate," *Journal of Speech and Hearing Disorders,* XVI (1951), 273-79.

87. _____ and D. C. Spriestersbach, "A Study of Minor Organic Deviations in Functional Disorders of Articulation: Rate of Movement of Oral Structures," *Journal of Speech and Hearing Disorders,* XV (1950), 60-69.

88. Fletcher, Harvey, *Speech and Hearing* (New York: D. Van Nostrand Co., 1929).

89. Fletcher, S. G., R. L. Casteel, and Doris P. Bradley, "Tongue-Thrust Swallow, Speech Articulation, and Age," *Journal of Speech and Hearing Disorders,* XXVI (1961).

90. Ford, Frank, *Diseases of the Nervous System in Infancy, Childhood and Adolescence,* 4th Ed. (Springfield, Ill.: Charles C Thomas, 1960).

91. Fox, Donna R., and Barbara S. McDonald, "Feeding Techniques: For Health and Speech," *Crippled Child,* XXXV (1958).

92. Froeschels, E., "A Practical Method for Checking Progress During the Treatment of Sigmatisms," *Practica Oto-Rhino-Laryngologica,* IX (1947), 358-64.

93. _____, "Chewing Method as Therapy," *Archives of Otolaryngology,* LVI (1952), 427-34.

94. _____, "Interdental Lisping and Multiple Interdentality on a Psychic Basis," *Practica Oto-Rhino-Laryngologica,* II (1939), 65-67.
95. _____, *Speech Therapy* (Magnolia, Mass.: Expression Co., 1933).
96. _____ and A. Jellinek, *Speech Therapy* (Magnolia, Mass.: Expression Co., 1941).
97. _____, S. Kastein, and D. A. Weiss, "A Method of Therapy for Paralytic Conditions of the Mechanisms of Phonation, Respiration and Glutination," *Journal of Speech and Hearing Disorders,* XX (1955).
98. Frowing, V. K., and H. Moser, "Relationship of Dentition and Speech," *Journal of American Dental Association,* XXXI (1944), 1001-90.
99. Fymbo, L. H., "The Relation of Malocclusion of the Teeth to Defects of Speech," *Archives of Speech,* I (1936), 204-16.
100. Gens, G., "The Speech Pathologist Looks at the Mentally Deficient Child," *Training School Bulletin,* LXVIII (1951), 19-27.
101. Gesell, A., and C. S. Amatruda, *Development Diagnosis: Normal and Abnormal Child Development* (New York: Paul B. Hoeber, Inc., 1941).
102. _____ et al., *Gesell Developmental Schedules* (New York: Psychological Corporation, 1949).
103. Glauber, P., "Speech Characteristics of Psychoneurotic Patients," *Journal of Speech and Hearing Disorders,* IX (1944), 18-30.
104. Goldman, Robert, and Macalyne Fristoe, "The Development of the Filmstrip Articulation Test," *Journal of Speech and Hearing Disorders,* XXXII (1967), 256-62.
105. Goldstein, Kurt, *Language and Language Disturbances* (New York: Grune and Stratton, 1948).
106. Goldstein, M. A., "Speech Without a Tongue," *Journal of Speech Disorders,* V (1940), 65-69.
107. Goodstein, L. D., "Functional Speech Disorders and Personality: A Survey of the Research," *Journal of Speech and Hearing Research,* I (1958).
108. Goodwin, F. B., "A Consideration of Etiologies in 454 Cases of Speech Retardation," *Journal of Speech and Hearing Disorders,* XX (1955).
109. Grewel, F., "Classification of Dysarthrias," *Acta Psychiatrica et Neurologica Scandinavica,* XXXII (1957).
110. Haas, William, "Phonological Analysis of a Case of Dyslalia," *Journal of Speech and Hearing Disorders,* XXVIII (1963), 239-46.
111. Hahn, E., "An Analysis of the Speech of First Grade Children," *Quarterly Journal of Speech,* XXXV (1949), 338-42.
112. Hall, M., "Auditory Factors in Functional Articulatory Speech Defects," *Journal of Experimental Education,* VII (1938), 110-32.
113. Hansen, B. F., "The Application of Sound Discrimination Tests to Functional Articulatory Defectives with Normal Hearing," *Journal of Speech Disorders,* IX (1944), 347-55.
114. Hardy, Janet B., Anne Dougherty, and W. G. Hardy, "Hearing Responses and Audiologic Screening in Infants," *Journal of Pediatrics,* LV (1959).
115. Hardy, William G., "On Language Disorders in Young Children: A

Reorganization of Thinking," *Journal of Speech and Hearing Disorders,* XXX (1965), 3-16.

116. Hawk, S. S., "Can a Child Be Taught to Talk?" *Journal of Speech Disorders,* IV (1939), 173-79.

117. _____, "Moto-Kinesthetic Speech Training for Children," *Journal of Speech Disorders,* II (1937), 231-37.

118. Head, Henry, *Aphasia and Kindred Disorders of Speech* (New York: The Macmillan Company, 1962).

119. Hebb, Donald O., *A Textbook of Psychology,* 2nd Ed. (Philadelphia: W. B. Saunders Co., 1966).

120. Hejna, R. F., *Developmental Articulation Test* (Ann Arbor, Mich.: Speech Materials, 1963).

121. Heltman, H. J., "Re-education Techniques in Speech Correction," *Journal of Speech Disorders,* I (1936), 41-46.

122. Henderson, F. M., "Accuracy in Testing the Articulation of Speech Sounds," *Journal of Educational Research,* XXXI (1937-38), 348-56.

123. Henrikson, E. H., "An Analysis of Wood's Articulation Index," *Journal of Speech and Hearing Disorders,* XIII (1948), 233-35.

124. Hilgard, Ernest K., *Introduction to Psychology,* 3rd Ed. (New York: Harcourt, Brace, and World, Inc., 1962).

125. Hixon, Thomas J., and James C. Hardy, "Restricted Motility of the Speech Articulators in Cerebral Palsy," *Journal of Speech and Hearing Disorders,* XXVIII (1964), 293-306.

126. Hoffman, Jeanette A., and Richard L. Hoffman, "Tongue-Thrust and Deglutition: Some Anatomical, Physiological, and Neurological Considerations," *Journal of Speech and Hearing Disorders,* XXX (1965), 105-20.

127. Hudgins, C. V., "A Comparative Study of the Speech Co-ordinations of Deaf and Normal Subjects," *Journal of Genetic Psychology,* XLIV (1934), 3-48.

128. _____, "Visual Aids in the Correction of Speech," *Volta Review,* XXXVII (1935), 637-43.

129. _____ and F. C. Numbers, "An Investigation of the Intelligibility of the Speech of the Deaf," *Genetic Psychology Monographs,* XXV (1942), 289-392.

130. Hull, M. E., "Anticipatory Speech Responses in Children with Articulation Defects," *Journal of Speech Disorders,* XIII (1948), 268-72.

131. Humphrey, W. R., and R. Milisen, "A Study of the Ability to Reproduce Unfamiliar Sounds which Have Been Presented Orally," *Journal of Speech and Hearing Disorders, Monograph Supplement,* No. 4 (1954), 57-70.

132. Irwin, J. V., and O. Becklund, "Norms for Maximum Repetitive Rates for Certain Sounds Established with the Sylrater," *Journal of Speech and Hearing Disorders,* XVIII (1953).

133. Irwin, O. C., "A Manual of Articulation Testing for Use with Children with Cerebral Palsy," *Cerebral Palsy Review,* XXII (1961).

134. _____, "Development of Speech During Infancy: Curve of Phonemic Frequencies" *Journal of Experimental Psychology,* XXXVII (1947), 187-93.

135. _____, "Infant Speech: Consonant Sounds According to Manner of Articulation," *Journal of Speech Disorders*, XII (1947), 402-4.

136. _____, "Infant Speech: Effect of Systematic Reading of Stories," *Journal of Speech and Hearing Research*, III (1960).

137. _____, "Infant Speech: Speech Sound Development of Sibling and Only Infants," *Journal of Experimental Psychology*, XXXVIII (1948).

138. _____, "Infant Speech: Variability and the Problem of Diagnosis," *Journal of Speech Disorders*, XII (1947).

139. _____ and H. P. Chen, "Development of Speech During Infancy: Curve of Phonemic Types," *Journal of Experimental Psychology*, XXXVI (1946).

140. Irwin, Ruth Beckey, "A Study of Certain Factors Related to Retardation of Speech," *Journal of Speech Disorders*, VII (1942), 223-49.

141. _____, *Speech and Hearing Therapy* (Englewood Cliffs, N.J.: Prentice-Hall, Inc., 1953).

142. _____ and Barbara W. Musselman "A Compact Picture Articulation Test," *Journal of Speech and Hearing Disorders*, XXVII (1962), 36-39.

143. Jackson, L., "Non-Speaking Children," *British Journal of Medical Psychology*, XXIII (1950), 87-100.

144. Jann, Gladys Reid, Marion Minst Ward, and Henry W. Jann, "Longitudinal Study of Articulation, Deglutition, and Malocclusion," *Journal of Speech and Hearing Disorders*, XXVIII (1964), 424-35.

145. _____ and Dorothea F. Whitman, *Lisping and Tongue Thrusting* (Penfield, N.Y.: Board of Cooperative Services, First Supervisory District of Monroe County, 1963).

146. Jenkins, Edna, and Frances E. Lohr, "Severe Articulation Disorders and Motor Ability," *Journal of Speech and Hearing Disorders*, XXVIII (1964), 286-92.

147. Johnson, Wendell, Spencer F. Brown, James F. Curtis, Clarence W. Edney, and Jacqueline Keaster, *Speech Handicapped School Children*, 3rd Ed. (New York: Harper & Row, Publishers, 1967).

148. _____, F. L. Darley, and D. C. Spriestersbach, *Diagnostic Methods in Speech Pathology* (New York: Harper & Row, Publishers, 1963).

149. Jones, Morris Val, *Baby Talk* (Springfield, Ill.: Charles C. Thomas, 1960).

150. Jordan, E. P., "Articulation Test Measures and Listener Ratings of Articulation Defectiveness," *Journal of Speech and Hearing Research*, III (1960).

151. Kanner, Leo, *Child Psychiatry*, 3rd Ed. (Springfield, Ill.: Charles C. Thomas, 1960).

152. Kaplan, Harold M., *Anatomy and Physiology of Speech* (New York: McGraw-Hill Book Co., 1960).

153. Karlin, I. W., A. C. Youta, and L. Kennedy, "Distorted Speech in Young Children," *American Journal of Diseases of Children*, LIX (1940), 1203-18.

154. Kenyon, John S., and Thomas A. Knott, *A Pronouncing Dictionary of American English* (Springfield, Mass.: G. and C. Merriam Co., 1953).

155. Kessler, H. E., "The Relationship of Dentistry to Speech," *Journal of American Dental Association*, XLVIII (1954), 44-49.

156. Kessler, Jane W., *The Psychopathology of Children* (Englewood Cliffs, N.J.: Prentice-Hall, Inc., 1966).

157. Knobel, H., "Relations Between Faulty Formation of Sibilants and Anomalies in the Placement of Upper Teeth," *Archiv für die gesamte Phonetic,* III (1939), 108-28.

158. Koepp-Baker, Herbert, *Handbook of Clinical Speech* (Ann Arbor, Mich.: Edwards Bros., 1936).

159. _____, "Palatomorphology of Cleft Palate and Cleft Lip," in *Handbook of Speech Pathology,* ed. L. E. Travis (New York: Appleton-Century-Crofts, Inc., 1957).

160. Krescheck, Jan Dawson, and John W. Black, "Appropriate Materials for Self-Administered Training in Intelligibility," *Journal of Speech and Hearing Disorders,* XXVIII (1964), 70-75.

161. Kronvall, E. L., and C. F. Diehl, "The Relationship of Auditory Discrimination to Articulation Defects of Children with No Known Organic Impairment," *Journal of Speech and Hearing Disorders* XIX (1954) 335-38.

162. Larr, A. L., *Tongue Thrust and Speech Correction* (San Francisco, Calif.: Fearon Publishers, 1962).

163. Leopold, W., *Speech Development of a Bilingual Child* (Evanston, Ill.: Northwestern University Press, 1947).

164. Lerea, L., "Assessing Language Development" *Journal of Speech and Hearing Research,* I (1958).

165. Lewis, James A., and Richard F. Counihan "Tongue-Thrust in Infancy," *Journal of Speech and Hearing Disorders,* XXX (1965), 280-82.

166. Lewis, M. M., *Infant Speech: A Study of the Beginnings of Language* (London: Routledge, & Kegan Paul, Ltd., 1951).

167. Lillywhite, Herold, "Make Mother a Clinician," *Journal of Speech Disorders,* XIII (1948), 61-66.

168. Lloyd, G. W., and S. Ainsworth, "The Classroom Teacher's Activities and Attitudes Relating to Speech Correction," *Journal of Speech and Hearing Disorders,* XIX (1954), 244-49.

169. Lloyd, M. P., *Our First Speech Book* (New York: Newsen and Co., 1942).

170. Luchsinger, R., and G. Arnold, *Voice-Speech-Language* (Belmont, Calif.: Wadsworth Publishing Co., Inc., 1965).

171. Lundeen, D. J., "The Relationship of Diadochokinesis to Various Speech Sounds," *Journal of Speech and Hearing Disorders,* XV (1950).

172. MacKeith, R., and M. Bax, *Minimal Cerebral Dysfunction* (London: William Heineman, Limited, 1963).

173. Mayer, P. McCullagh, and Wilson A. Swanker, *Anomalies of Infants and Children* (New York: McGraw-Hill Book Company, Inc., 1958).

174. McCarthy, Dorothea, "Language Development in Children," in *Manual of Child Psychology,* ed. L. Charmichael (New York: John Wiley & Sons, Inc., 1954).

175. _____, "Some Possible Explanations of Sex Differences in Language Development and Disorders," *Journal of Psychology,* XXXV (1953).

176. _____, *The Language Development of the Preschool Child, Child Welfare Monograph, No. 4* (Minneapolis: University of Minnesota Press, 1930).

177. McCarthy, J. J., and S. A. Kirk, *Illinois Test of Psycholinguistic Abilities: Examiner's Manual* (Urbana: University of Illinois Institute for Research on Exceptional Children, 1961).

178. McCrosky Robert L., "Some Effects of Anesthetizing the Articulators Under Conditions of Normal and Delayed Side Tone," U.S. Naval School of Aviation Medicine. Pensacola, Fla., Project NM 001 104 500, Report No. 65, 1956.

179. McCurry, W. H., and O. C. Irwin, "A Study of Word Approximations in the Spontaneous Speech of Infants," *Journal of Speech and Hearing Disorders*, XVIII (1953), 133-39.

180. McDonald, Eugene, *Articulation Testing and Treatment: A Sensory-Motor Approach* (Pittsburgh, Penn.: Stanwix House, Inc., 1964).

181. _____ and Burton Chance, Jr., *Cerebral Palsy* (Englewood Cliffs, N.J.: Prentice-Hall, Inc., 1964).

182. McWilliams, Betty Jane, "Articulation Problems in a Group of Cleft Palate Adults," *Journal of Speech and Hearing Research*, I (1958).

183. Marge, Dorothy K., "The Social Status of Speech-Handicapped Children," *Journal of Speech and Hearing Research*, IX (1966), 165-77.

184. Mase, D. J., *Etiology of Articulatory Speech Defects* (New York: Columbia University Teacher's College Contributions to Education, No. 921, 1946).

185. Matthews, Jack, "Speech Problems of the Mentally Retarded," in *Handbook of Speech Pathology*, ed. L. E. Travis (New York: Appleton-Century-Crofts, Inc., 1957).

186. Mead, C. D., "The Age of Walking and Talking in Relation to General Intelligence," *Pedagogical Seminary*, XX (1913), 460-84.

187. Mecham, M. J., *Verbal Language Development Scale* (Minneapolis, Minn.: American Guidance Service, 1959).

188. _____, M. J. Berko, and F. G. Berko, *Speech Therapy in Cerebral Palsy* (Springfield, Ill.: Charles C Thomas, 1960).

189. Metraux, R. W., "Auditory Memory Span for Speech Sounds: Norms for Children," *Journal of Speech Disorders*, IX (1944), 31-38.

190. _____, "Speech Profiles of the Pre-School Child 18 to 54 Months," *Journal of Speech and Hearing Disorders*, XV (1950), 37-53.

191. Mikalsen, E., *Speech Development Records for Children* (Pasadena, Calif.: Pacific Records Distributing Co., Box 2038-D).

192. Milisen, R., "The Disorders of Articulation: A Systematic Clinical and Experimental Approach," *Journal of Speech and Hearing Disorders, Monograph Supplement, No. 4* (1954).

193. _____, "The Incidence of Speech Disorders," in *Handbook of Speech Pathology*, ed. L. E. Travis (New York: Appleton-Century-Crofts, Inc., 1957).

194. _____, "Methods of Evaluation and Diagnosis of Speech Disorders," in *Handbook of Speech Pathology*, ed. L. E. Travis (New York: Appleton-Century-Crofts, Inc., 1957).

195. Mims, Howard A., Christy Kolas, and Ronald Williams, "Lisping and Persistent Thumb-Sucking among Children with Open-Bite Malocclusions," *Journal of Speech and Hearing Disorders*, XXXI (1966), 176-77.

196. Moll, K. L., and F. L. Darley, "Attitudes of Mothers of Articulatory-Impaired and Speech-Retarded Children," *Journal of Speech and Hearing Disorders,* XXV (1960).

197. Monrad-Krohn, G. H., "Dysprosody or Altered 'Melody of Language,' " *Brain,* LXX (1947).

198. Morley, D. E., "The Rehabilitation of Adults with Dysarthric Speech," *Journal of Speech and Hearing Disorders,* XX (1955).

199. Morley, Muriel, *Cleft Palate and Speech,* 6th Ed. (Baltimore, Md.: The Williams & Wilkins Company, 1966).

200. _____, *Development and Disorders of Speech in Childhood,* 2nd Ed. (Baltimore, Md.: Williams & Wilkins Company, 1965).

201. _____, D. Court, and H. Miller, "Developmental Dysarthria," *British Medical Journal,* I (1954), 8-12.

202. Morris, H. L., D. C. Spriestersbach, and F. L. Darley, "An Articulation Test for Assessing Competency of Velopharyngeal Closure," *Journal of Speech and Hearing Research,* IV (1961).

203. Morrison, S., "Measuring the Severity of Articulation Defectiveness," *Journal of Speech and Hearing Disorders,* XX (1955), 347-51.

204. Mosher, J. A., *The Production of Correct Speech Sounds* (Magnolia, Mass.: Expression Co., 1929).

205. Mowrer, O. H., "Speech Development in the Young Child: 1. The Autism Theory of Speech Development and Some Clinical Applications," *Journal of Speech and Hearing Disorders,* XXVII (1952), 263-68.

206. Mussen, Paul H., John J. Conger, and Jerome Kagan, *Readings in Child Development and Personality* (New York: Harper & Row, Publishers, 1965).

207. Myklebust, H., *Auditory Disorders in Children* (New York: Grune & Stratton, 1954).

208. Mysak, Edward D., "Dysarthria and Oropharyngeal Reflexology: A Review," *Journal of Speech and Hearing Disorders,* XXVIII (1963), 252-60.

209. _____, *Speech Pathology and Feedback Theory* (Springfield, Ill.: Charles C Thomas, 1966).

210. Nathanson, Y. S., and J. E. Nathanson, *Manual of Corrective Speech Exercises* (Philadelphia: J. Nathanson, 1947).

211. Nemoy, E. M., *Speech Correction Through Story Telling Units* (Magnolia. Mass.: Expression Co., 1954).

212. _____ and S. Davis, *The Correction of Defective Consonant Sounds* (Magnolia, Mass.: Expression Co., 1937).

213. Newby, Hayes, *Audiology* (New York: Appleton-Century-Crofts, Inc., 1958).

214. Nielsen, J. M., *Agnosia, Apraxia, Aphasia,* 2nd Ed. (New York: Paul B. Hoeber, Inc., 1947).

215. Ogilvie, M., *Terminology and Definitions of Speech Defects* (New York: Teacher's College, Columbia University Contributions to Education, No. 859, 1942).

216. O'Neill John J., *The Hard of Hearing* (Englewood Cliffs, N.J.: Prentice-Hall, Inc., 1964).

217. Orton, S. T., *Reading, Writing, and Speech Problems in Children* (New York: W. W. Norton and Company, Inc., 1937).

218. Osgood, C. E., and S. M. Miron, *Approaches to the Study of Aphasia* (Chicago: University of Chicago Press, 1962).

219. Palmer, John M., "Tongue Thrusting: A Clinical Hypothesis," *Journal of Speech and Hearing Disorders*, XXVII (1964), 323-33.

220. _____ and Dominic LaRusso, *Anatomy for Speech and Hearing* (New York: Harper & Row, Publishers, 1965).

221. Peacher, W. G., "Neurological Factors in Etiology of Delayed Speech," *Journal of Speech and Hearing Disorders*, XIV (1949).

222. _____, "The Etiology and Differential Diagnosis of Dysarthria," *Journal of Speech and Hearing Disorders*, XV (1950), 252-65.

223. Penfield, Wilder, and T. Rasmussen, *The Cerebral Cortex of Man* (New York: The Macmillan Co., 1950).

224. _____ and Lamar Roberts, *Speech and Brain Mechanisms* (Princeton, N.J.: Princeton University Press, 1959).

225. Peppard, H., *The Correction of Speech Defects* (New York: The Macmillan Co., 1925).

226. Perlstein, M. A., and E. T. McDonald, "Nature, Recognition and Management of Neuromuscular Disabilities in Children," *Pediatrics*, XI (1953).

227. Perrin, E. L., "The Rating of Defective Speech by Trained and Untrained Observers," *Journal of Speech and Hearing Disorders*, XIX (1954), 48-51.

228. Poole, I., "Genetic Development of Articulation of Consonant Sounds in Speech," *Elementary English Review*, XI (1934), 159-61.

229. Powers, Margaret H., "Clinical and Educational Procedures in Functional Disorders of Articulation" *Handbook of Speech Pathology*, ed. L. E. Travis (New York: Appleton-Century-Crofts, Inc., 1957).

230. _____, "Functional Disorders of Articulation—Symptomatology and Etiology," *Handbook of Speech Pathology*, ed. L. E. Travis (New York: Appleton-Century-Crofts, Inc., 1957).

231. Prins, David, "Relations among Specific Articulatory Deviations and Responses to a Clinical Measure of Sound Discrimination Ability," *Journal of Speech and Hearing Disorders*, XXVIII (1963), 382-88.

232. Pronovost, W., "Visual Aids to Speech Improvement," *Journal of Speech Disorders*, XII (1947), 387-91.

233. _____ and C. Dumbelton, "A Picture Type Speech Sound Discrimination Test," *Journal of Speech and Hearing Disorders*, XVIII (1953), 258-66.

234. Raph, Jane Beasley, "Language and Speech Deficits in Culturally Disadvantaged Children, and Their Implications for the Speech Clinician," *Journal of Speech and Hearing Disorders*, XXXII (1967), 203-14.

235. Raubicheck, L., in McDowell, E., "The Role of Speech Training in a Program of Orthodontic Treatment," *International Journal of Orthodontia and Oral Surgery*, XXII (1936), 110-13.

236. Reid, G., "The Efficacy of Speech Re-education of Functional Articulatory Defects in Elementary School Children," *Journal of Speech Disorders*, XII (1947), 363-68.

237. ———, "The Etiology and Nature of Functional Articulatory Defects in Elementary School Children," *Journal of Speech Disorders,* XII (1947), 143-50.

238. Ringel, Robert L., "Some Effects of Tactile and Auditory Alterations on Speech Output," Doctoral Dissertation, Purdue University, 1962.

239. Robbins, S. D., "Aids in Correcting Articulatory Defects," *Proceedings of American Speech Correction Association,* IV (1934), 22-31.

240. ———, "Importance of Sensory Training in Speech Therapy," *Journal of American Speech Correction Association,* VII (1942), 183-88.

241. ———, "The Relation Between the Short Auditory Memory Disability and Disorders of Speech," *Proceedings of American Society for Study of Disorders of Speech,* III (1932), 9-15.

242. ——— and S. M. Stichfield, *Dictionary of Terms Dealing with Disorders of Speech* (Magnolia, Mass.: Expression Co., 1931).

243. Roe, Vivian, and R. L. Milisen, "The Effect of Maturation upon Defective Articulation in Elementary Grades," *Journal of Speech Disorders,* VII (1942).

244. Roman, E. F., and R. Milisen, "Effect of Latency Between Stimulation and Response on Reproduction of Sounds," *Journal of Speech and Hearing Disorders, Monograph Supplement, No. 4* (1954), 71-79.

245. Ronson, Irwin, "Incidence of Visceral Swallow among Lispers," *Journal of Speech and Hearing Disorders,* XXX (1965), 318-24.

246. Rose, J. A., "Dynamics and Treatment of Speech Disorders," *American Journal of Orthopsychiatry,* XIII (1943), 284-89.

247. Round, H., "Oral and Facial Restorations in Connection with Speech Defects," *Speech* (London), II (1936), 19-38.

248. Rubin, Herbert Asher Bar, and John H. Dwyer, "An Experimental Speech and Language Program for Psychotic Children," *Journal of Speech and Hearing Disorders,* XXXII (1967), 242-48.

249. Rutherford, Berneice, *Give Them A Chance to Talk* (Minneapolis, Minn.: Burgess Publishing Co., 1956).

250. Safier, D. E., *The Listening Book* (Caldwell, Idaho: The Caxton Printers, 1952).

251. Sale, M., and Joseph M. Wepman, "A Screening Survey of Organic Impairment," *Journal of Speech Disorders,* X (1945), 283-86.

252. Sanford, Fillmore, *Psychology: A Scientific Study of Man* (Belmont, Calif.: Wadsworth Publishing Co., Inc., 1965).

253. ———, "Speech and Personality," *Psychological Bulletin,* XXXIX (1942), 811-45.

254. Saunders, M. J., "The Short Auditory Memory Span Disability," *Childhood Education,* VIII (1931), 59-66.

255. Sayler, H. K., "The Effect of Maturation upon Defective Articulation in Grades Seven through Twelve," *Journal of Speech and Hearing Disorders,* XIV (1949), 202-7.

256. Schiefelbusch, R. L., *et al.,* "Language Studies of Mentally Retarded Children," *Journal of Speech and Hearing Disorders, Monograph Supplement, No. 10* (1963).

257. Schlanger, B. B., "Speech Measurements of Institutionalized Mentally Handicapped Children." *American Journal of Mental Deficiency,* LVIII (1953), 114-22.

258. ———, "Speech Therapy Results with Mentally Retarded Children in Special Classes," *Training School Bulletin,* L (1953), 179-86.

259. Schlesinger, Bruno, *Higher Cerebral Functions and Their Clinical Disorders* (New York: Grune and Stratton, 1962).

260. Schneider, B., and J. Vallen, "A Speech Therapy Program for Mentally Retarded Children," *American Journal of Mental Deficiency,* LVIII (1954), 633-39.

261. Schneiderman, Norma, "A Study of the Relationship Between Articulatory Ability and Language Ability," *Journal of Speech and Hearing Disorders,* XX (1955).

262. Schuell, Hildred, "Aphasic Difficulties in Understanding Spoken Language," *Neurology,* III (1953).

263. ———, James J. Jenkins, Edward Jiminez-Pabon, *Aphasia in Adults* (New York: Harper & Row, Publishers, 1964).

264. Scott, D. A., and R. Milisen, "The Effectiveness of Combined Visual, Auditory and Combined Visual-Auditory Stimulation upon the Speech Responses of Defective Speaking Children." *Journal of Speech and Hearing Disorders, Monograph Supplement, No. 4* (1954), 37-44.

265. ———, and R. Milisen, "The Effectiveness of Combined Visual-Auditory Stimulation in Improving Articulation," *Journal of Speech and Hearing Disorders, Monograph Supplement, No. 4* (1954), 51-56.

266. Scripture, E. W., *Stuttering, Lisping and Correction of the Speech of the Deaf* (New York: The Macmillan Co., 1926).

267. Searl, N., "Some Emotional Factors Affecting Children's Speech," *Speech* (London), II (1935), 21-29.

268. Seth, G., and D. Guthrie, *Speech in Childhood* (London: Oxford University Press, 1935).

269. Shames, G., "An Investigation of Prognosis and Evaluation in Speech Therapy," *Journal of Speech and Hearing Disorders,* XVII (1952), 386-92.

270. Shelton, Ralph L., Alta R. Brooks, and Karl A. Youngstrom, "Articulation and Patterns of Palatopharyngeal Closure," *Journal of Speech and Hearing Disorders,* XXVIII (1964), 390-408.

271. ———, Alta R. Brooks, and Karl A. Youngstrom, "Clinical Assessment of Palatopharyngeal Closure," *Journal of Speech and Hearing Disorders,* XXX (1965), 37-43.

272. Sherman, Dorothy, and S. Morrison, "Reliability of Individual Ratings of Severity of Defective Articulation," *Journal of Speech and Hearing Disorders,* XX (1955), 352-58.

273. ———, and Annette Geith, "Speech Sound Discrimination and Articulation Skill," *Journal of Speech and Hearing Research,* X (1967), 277-80.

274. Siegel, Gerald M., "Experienced and Inexperienced Articulation Examiners," *Journal of Speech and Hearing Disorders,* XXVIII (1962).

275. ———, Harris Winitz, and Harlan Conkey, "The Influence of Testing Instrument on Articulatory Responses in Children," *Journal of Speech and Hearing Disorders,* XXVIII (1963), 67-76.

276. Simon, Clarence T., "The Development of Speech," in *Handbook of Speech Pathology,* ed. L. E. Travis (New York: Appleton-Century-Crofts, Inc., 1957).

277. Simonson, Josephone, "Speech as a Diagnostic Aid," in *Common Neurologic Problems. Medical Clinics of North America*, 44, 1960.

278. Smith, Madorah E., "Some Light on the Problem of Bilingualism as Found from a Study of the Progress in Mastery of English among Pre-school Children of Non-American Ancestry in Hawaii," *Genetic Psychology Monographs*, XXI (1939).

279. Smith, S., "The Influence of Illness During the First Two Years of Infant Development," *Journal of Genetic Psychology*, XXXIX (1931), 284-87.

280. Snow, Katherine, "Articulation Proficiency in Relation to Certain Dental Abnormalities," *Journal of Speech and Hearing Disorders*, XXVI (1961).

281. _____ and R. Milisen, "The Influence of Oral Versus Pictorial Presentation upon Articulation Testing Results," *Journal of Speech and Hearing Disorders, Monograph Supplement, No. 4* (1954), 29-36.

282. Sommers, Ronald K., Ann K. Furlong, Frank E. Rhodes, George R. Fichter, Delores C. Bowser, Florence G. Copetas, and Zane G. Saunders, "Effects of Maternal Attitudes upon Improvement in Articulation when Mothers are Trained to Assist in Speech Correction," *Journal of Speech and Hearing Disorders*, XXVIII (1964), 126-32.

283. _____, Morton H. Schaeffer, Robert H. Leiss, Adele J. Gerber, Mary Ann Bray, Delores Fundrella, Janice K. Olson, and Elizabeth R. Tomkins. "The Effectiveness of Group and Individual Therapy," *Journal of Speech and Hearing Research*, IX (1966), 219-25.

284. Spiker, C. C., and O. C. Irwin, "The Relationship Between I.Q. and Indices of Infant Speech Sound Development," *Journal of Speech and Hearing Disorders*, XIV (1949).

285. Spriestersbach, D. C., "Counseling Parents of Children with Cleft Lips and Palates," *Journal of Chronic Diseases*, XIII (1961).

286. _____ and J. Curtis, "Misarticulation and Discrimination of Speech Sounds," *Quarterly Journal of Speech*, XXXVII (1951), 483-91.

287. St. Onge, K., "Brain Damage Syndrome: Speech and Psychological Factors," *Journal of Speech and Hearing Disorders*, XXIV (1959), 43-50.

288. Stasney, R., "Parent Counseling in Speech Correction," *Western Speech*, XV (1951), 17-22.

289. Steer, M. D., and Hazel G. Drexler, "Predicting Later Articulation Ability from Kindergarten Tests," *Journal of Speech and Disorders*, XXV (1960).

290. Stein, L., *The Infancy of Speech and the Speech of Infancy* (London: Methuen & Co., Ltd., 1947).

291. Stern, E., "Recent Research in Dyslalias," *Journal of Logopaedics*, I (1937), 26-31.

292. Stetson, R. H., *Motor Phonetics*, 2nd Ed. (Oberlin, O.: Oberlin College, 1951).

293. Stinchfield, S. M., and Edna Hill Young, *Children with Delayed or Defective Speech* (Palo Alto, Calif.: Stanford University Press, 1938).

294. _____ and Edna Hill Young, *The Moto-Kinesthetic Method of Speech Training* (Palo Alto, Calif.: Stanford University Press, 1955).

295. Strauss, A. A., and Laura Lehtinen, *Psychopathology and Education of the Brain-Injured Child* (New York: Grune and Stratton, 1950).

296. ———— and N. C. Kephart, *Psychopathology and Education of the Brain-Injured Child,* Vol. 2 (New York: Grune and Stratton, 1955).

297. Streng, Alice, Waring J. Fitch, LeRoy D. Hedgecock, James W. Phillips, and James A. Carrell, *Hearing Therapy for Children* (New York: Grune and Stratton, 1955).

298. Subtelny, Joanne D., Jorge C. Mestre, and J. Daniel Subtelny, "Comparative Study of Normal and Defective Articulation of /s/ as Related to Malocclusion and Deglutition," *Journal of Speech and Hearing Disorders,* XXVIII (1964), 269-85.

299. Sullivan, E. M., "Auditory Acuity and Its Relation to Defective Speech, *Journal of Speech Disorders,* IX (1944), 127-30.

300. Summers, R., "Perceptive vs. Productive Skills in Analyzing Speech Sounds from Words," *Journal of Speech and Hearing Disorders,* XVIII (1953), 140-48.

301. Taylor, John R., "Screening Intelligence," *Journal of Speech and Hearing Disorders,* XXVIII (1963), 90-91.

302. Tattersfield, A., "The Speech and Language of the Pre-School Child," *Speech* (London), XVI (1952), 8-20.

303. Templin, Mildred C., "A Non-Diagnostic Articulation Test," *Journal of Speech Disorders,* XII (1947), 392-96.

304. ————, "A Study of the Sound Discriminability of Elementary School Pupils," *Journal of Speech Disorders,* VIII (1943), 127-32.

305. ————, *Certain Language Skills in Children: Their Development and Interrelationships, Child Welfare Monographs, No. 26* (Minneapolis, Minn.: University of Minnesota Press, 1957).

306. ————, "Norms on a Screening Test of Articulation for Ages Three Through Eight," *Journal of Speech and Hearing Disorders,* XVIII (1953), 323-31.

307. ————, "Spontaneous Versus Imitated Verbalization in Testing Articulation in Pre-School Children," *Journal of Speech Disorders,* XII (1947), 293-300.

308. ———— and M. D. Steer, "Studies of Growth of Speech of Pre-School Children," *Journal of Speech Disorders,* IV (1939), 71-77.

309. Tizard, J. P. M., R. S. Paine, and B. Crothers, "Disturbances of Sensation in Children with Hemiplegia," *Journal of the American Medical Association,* CLV (1954).

310. Trager, G., L., and H. L. Smith, *An Outline of English Structure* (Washington, D.C.: American Council of Learned Societies, 1957).

311. Travis, L. E., *Speech Pathology* (New York: Appleton-Century-Crofts, Inc., 1931).

312. ————, "The Pedagogical Significance of the Moto-Kinesthetic Method in Speech Therapy," *Journal of Speech Disorders,* V (1940), 281-84.

313. ———— and B. Rasmus, "The Speech Sound Discrimination Ability of Cases with Functional Disorders of Articulation," *Quarterly Journal of Speech,* XVII (1937), 217-26.

314. ———— and LaVerne Deel Sutherland, "Suggestions for Psychotherapy in Public School Speech Correction," in *Handbook of Speech Pathology,* ed. L. E. Travis (New York: Appleton-Century-Crofts, Inc., 1957).

315. Trim, J. L. M., "Some Suggestions for the Phonetic Notation of Sounds in Defective Speech," *Speech* (London), XVII (1953), 21-24.
316. Twitmeyer, E. B., and Y. S. Nathanson, *Correction of Defective Speech* (New York: McGraw-Hill Book Company, 1932).
317. Utley, J., "The Relationship Between Speech Sound Discrimination and Percentage of Hearing Loss," *Journal of Speech Disorders,* IX (1944), 103-13.
318. Van Riper, Charles, *Speech Correction, Principles and Methods,* 4th Ed. (Englewood Cliffs, N.J.: Prentice-Hall, Inc., 1963).
319. _____, "Success and Failure in Speech Therapy." *Journal of Speech and Hearing Disorders,* XXXI (1966), 276-78.
320. _____ and John V. Irwin, *Voice and Articulation* (Englewood Cliffs, N.J.: Prentice-Hall, Inc., 1958).
321. Van Thal, J. H., "Tongue Thrusting in Relation to Sigmatism," *Speech* (London), XVIII (1954), 1-3.
322. Voelker, C. H., "Incidence of Pathologic Speech Behavior in the American General Population," *Archives of Otolaryngology,* XXXVIII (1933), 113-21.
323. Ward, Ida, *Defects of Speech: Their Nature and Their Cure* (New York: E. P. Dutton and Co., 1923).
324. *Webster's Third New International Dictionary of the English Language* (Springfield, Mass.; G. and C. Merriam Co., 1966).
325. Webster, Elizabeth J., "Parent Counseling by Speech Pathologists and Audiologists," *Journal of Speech and Hearing Disorders,* XXXI (1966), 331-40.
326. _____, William H. Perkins, H. Harlan Bloomer, and Wilbert Pronovost, "Case Selection in the Schools," *Journal of Speech and Hearing Disorders,* XXXI (1966), 352-58.
327. Weiss, D. A., "Organic Lesions Leading to Speech Disorders," *Nervous Child,* VII (1948), 29-37.
328. _____, "Speech Retarded Children," *Nervous Child,* IX (1951), 21-30.
329. Wellman, B. L., I. Case, I. Mengert, and D. Bradbury, "Speech Sounds of Young Children," *University of Iowa Studies in Child Welfare,* V (1931).
330. Wepman, Joseph, *Auditory Discrimination Test* (Chicago: 950 E. 59th Street, 1958).
331. West, Robert, M. Ansberry, and Anna Carr, *The Rehabilitation of Speech,* 3rd Ed. (New York: Harper & Row, Publishers, 1957).
332. _____, "The Neurophysiology of Speech," in *Handbook of Speech Pathology,* ed. L. E. Travis (New York: Appleton-Century-Crofts. Inc., 1957).
333. Westlake, Harold, *A System for Developing Speech with Cerebral Palsied Children* (Chicago: National Society for Crippled Children and Adults, Inc., 1952).
334. _____ and David R. Rutherford, *Cleft Palate* (Englewood Cliffs, N.J.: Prentice-Hall, Inc., 1966).
335. _____ and David R. Rutherford, *Speech Therapy for the Cerebral Palsied* (Chicago: National Society for Crippled Children and Adults, Inc., 1961).
336. Wilson, Frank B., "Efficacy of Speech Therapy with Educable Men-

tally Retarded Children," *Journal of Speech and Hearing Research,* IX (1966), 423-33.

337. Winitz, Harris, "Temporal Reliability in Articulation Testing," *Journal of Speech and Hearing Disorders,* XXVIII (1963), 247-51.

338. Wise, Claude M., *Applied Phonetics* (Englewood Cliffs, N.J.: Prentice-Hall, Inc., 1957).

339. Wolf, I. J., "The Relation of Malocclusion to Sigmatism," *American Journal of Diseases of Children,* LIV (1937), 520-28.

340. Wolpe, Zelda S., "Play Therapy, Psychodrama, and Parent Counseling," in *Handbook of Speech Pathology,* ed. L. E. Travis (New York: Appleton-Century-Crofts, Inc., 1957).

341. Wood, Kenneth S., "Measurement of Progress in the Correction of Articulatory Speech Defects," *Journal of Speech and Hearing Disorders,* XIV (1949).

342. _____, "Parental Maladjustment and Functional Articulatory Defects in Children," *Journal of Speech Disorders,* XI (1946), 255-75.

343. _____, "Terminology and Nomenclature," in *Handbook of Speech Pathology,* ed. L. E. Travis (New York: Appleton-Century-Crofts, Inc., 1957).

344. Wood, Nancy S., *Language Disorders in Children* (Chicago: National Society for Crippled Children and Adults, Inc., 1959).

345. _____, *Delayed Speech and Language Development* (Englewood Cliffs, N.J.: Prentice-Hall, Inc., 1964).

346. Woodburne, Lloyd S., *The Neural Basis of Behavior* (Columbus, O.: Charles E. Merrill Books, Inc., 1967).

347. Wright, A. K., "The Effect of Maternal Attitudes on the Outcome of Treatment of Children's Speech Defects," *Smith College Studies in Social Work,* X (1939), 123-24.

348. Wright, H. N., "Reliability of Evaluations During Basic Articulation and Stimulation Testing," *Journal of Speech and Hearing Disorders, Monograph Supplement, No. 4* (1954), 20-27.

349. Wyllie, J., *Disorders of Speech* (Edinburgh: Oliver and Boyd, 1894).

350. Young, Edna Hill, "Moto-Kinesthetic Approach to the Prevention of Speech Defects, Including Stuttering," *Journal of Speech and Hearing Disorders,* XXX (1965), 269-73.

351. Zaliouk, A., "A Visual-Tactile System of Phonetical Symbolization," *Journal of Speech and Hearing Disorders,* XIX (1954), 190-207.

352. Zimbardo, Philip G., George F. Mahl, and James W. Barnard, "Measurement of Speech Disturbance in Anxious Children," *Journal of Speech and Hearing Disorders,* XXVIII (1963), 362-70.

353. Zisk, Paulette Kendler, and Irv Bailer, "Speech and Language Problems in Mongolism: A Review of the Literature," *Journal of Speech and Hearing Disorders,* XXXII (1967), 228-41.

index

index